witness to pain

witness to pain

essays on the translation of pain into art

nieves pascual, ed.

PETER LANG
Bern · Berlin · Bruxelles · Frankfurt am Main · New York · Oxford · Wien

Bibliographic information published by Die Deutsche Bibliothek
Die Deutsche Bibliothek lists this publication in the Deutsche Nationalbibliografie; detailed bibliographic data is available on the Internet at ‹http://dnb.ddb.de›.

British Library and Library of Congress Cataloguing-in-Publication Data:
A catalogue record for this book is available from *The British Library,* Great Britain, and from *The Library of Congress,* USA

ISBN 3-03910-587-6
US-ISBN 0-8204-7041-4

Hochfeldstrasse 32, Postfach 746, CH-3000 Bern 9, Switzerland
info@peterlang.com, www.peterlang.com, www.peterlang.net

Printed in Germany

Table of Contents

III. Contagion through Looking

Introduction

To Schopenhauer the aim of life is pain. Pain is the norm, he writes (17). Pain to him gives sense to our existence because without pain we would be incapable of experiencing pleasure. Certainly, pain is not an exceptional experience. Most people have suffered or will suffer acute pain. To Hans-Georg Gadamer, in fact, we are all patients (98). It is also true that without pain there is no pleasure. But pain is not everyone's purpose in life. It is only when pain is given a purpose and becomes meaningful that life can go on. To Boris Cyrulnik in his treatise on resilience it is only when pain, or the memory of it, can be turned into art that it is bearable (13–14).

As it is, different purposes have served the reality of pain across history. On the one hand, it has been translated as a means to salvation and knowledge. On the other, it has been conceived of as a source of inspiration and artistic creation. In fact, Augustine, Joyce, Freud, Virginia Woolf, Shelley, Keats, Mansfield, Stevenson, Nietzsche, Jaspers, Kafka, Proust, Leopardi, Balzac, Juan Ramón Jiménez, Alberti, Aleixandre and others considered that it was needed to be industrious. However, it has also been coded as an indicator of moral corruption and punishment. Unfortunately, the idea of pain as guilt is still ingrained within us, even more so when physical suffering is caused by an illness stigmatised by society and culture. Be that as it may, pain inevitably effects a change of self that requires authentication by way of art because, eventually, it is the representation of pain, not pain itself, that persists in memory. Grünewald, Stanzione, Munch, Bacon, Bergman, Eisensten, Goya and Khalo have all attempted to represent the reality of pain, and yet they all have resigned themselves to evoke its idea because pain is too literal to allow representation.

Inevitably the art of pain comes from a witness, i.e., a doctor, an ex-patient or an onlooker sympathetic with the pain of the other. According to Arthur W. Frank, in the modern period pain was the prerogative of medicine (15). Narratives and photographs mapped the trajectory of disease and assigned causes and effects to the human body's symptoms. All of them followed a rigid set of prescriptions that increased efficacy but deprived the patients of agency.

In the wake of poststructuralism we witness an increase of individuation that results in an increase of pain autobiographies. Former patients, now recovered from intense pain, gain their language back and resort to art so as to counterbalance the little scope for agency felt during the illness. Whatever medium they choose to convey their experience, the shape of their story is, as Frank argues, 'moulded by all the rhetorical expectations that the storyteller has been internalising ever since he first heard some relative describe the illness, or she saw the first television commercial for a non-prescription remedy [...]. From [...] families and friends, from the popular culture that surrounds them, and from the stories of other ill people' (3). It follows that pain is socially constructed. Culture teaches us how to apprehend and suffer pain and indoctrinates the kind of story and meaning we must attach to it. Consequently, pain is portrayed differently in different parts of the world, but within one social space the same metaphors and conventions recur to describe its reality. This uniformity occludes the possibility of a private language in situations of pain and erodes the therapeutic implications usually assigned to art. If for art to be a health initiative the artist must of necessity carve a new language, as Deleuze argues (14), the art of pain may not relieve the symptoms. Furthermore, by bringing pain to consciousness art might even propitiate the re-enactment of the experience.

The third type of witness is the onlooker who sympathizes with the sufferer and presents the story of his/her viewing. Mary Ann Doane has theorized the concept of sympathy as a physiological one that 'connotes a process of contagion within the body, or between bodies' (172). If this is so, through sympathy contagion might occur. If by looking you might simulate an illness and contract some of the symptoms, the possibility of appropriating the pain of the other, which eventually becomes yours, is excluded.

This book is accordingly divided into three sections that necessarily overlap. In 'Strategies of Medical Discourse' attention is paid to clinical protocol. In his piece of autobiographical criticism, Mark Mossman examines the language used by doctors to describe his end-stage renal disease, and explains how despite his efforts to resist its engulfing effects, he eventually chooses to submit. Yet, his is a forced choice because the medical industry, he declares, 'wrecks those individuals who try to have some volition in the development of the meaning of their own lives. Medicine does not treat illness!', he claims with vehemence, but rather, '[I]t constructs reality itself in the attempt to structure and re-structure the "ill" body'. In this line of reasoning, Ángel Cagigas illustrates how Jean-Martin Charcot cured at the Salpêtrière the illness that he had created, cultivated and disseminated by means of aestheticized pictures. Focusing on photographs, the third essay analyses the work of several artists who have performed their breast cancer in the attempt to take control of their bodies. However, in mimicking surgery photographs some of them inevitably transform their bodies into symptoms and re-inscribe past wounds.

The second part, 'Restor(y)ing Pain through Life-Narratives' centres on the purposes of pain and its performances. Dana Milstein in 'Pain is a Preposition' argues that the simulation of pain by way of art is required to re-form identity and re-establish authority over one's own life. Whether reduplicated to inspire compassion, give rise to empathy, or engage the audience in the process of suffering, pain is a vehicle for the production of art. As it happens, only in the vulnerability of the body in pain is the subject capable of profound meditation. So, pain stimulates the process of creation, which in itself is a painful act of dispossession that paradoxically registers, in Summers-Bremmer's view, as a pleasurable gain. It momentarily satisfies the desire for pain and art, but does not extinguish it. In fact, it cannot extinguish desire because, as Bergman justifies in her analysis of Lars Gustafasson's *Death of a Beekeeper*, our private pain cannot be grasped with our tools of logic. To contain it with words would involve the dissolution of suffering and the death of art.

In the light of Locke's and Beccaria's theories, Valerie de Courville concentrates on the onlookers of pain, and shows that by exciting its idea the Gothic novel brings about the elevation of the spectators' soul and increases the efficacy of governmental control. The argument is shared by Markus Rheindorf, who analyses the role of pain in mainstream action films and the effects it triggers in the bodies of the audience. Departing from a Deleuzean view of the body as a site of intensities, he debates that pain has a deterritorializing effect that hardens and reaffirms pre-existing social structures. This third section on 'Contagion through Looking' concludes with an essay by Capeloa Gil in which she examines how the tragedy of Medea, the dismembering of her brother and the beheading of her two sons at her own hands is figured by Robinson Jeffers (1946) and George Tabori (1984). She comes to the conclusion that whereas the former uses transgression to legitimate traditional strategies, the latter subverts the myth, creating a simulacrum of Medea.

Pain is a hieroglyph. It liquidates the individual, but, within the same movement, it confers identity. Its enactment gives you agency, but deprives you of agency in a culture that demands a narrative when you are in pain and instructs you on the sensation terms to use. The art of pain is said to be therapeutic, but it could also void the self of self and become re-traumatizing. The pain of the other is incommensurable but you can understand it by making it yours. All these paradoxes and new ones are discovered here.

Works Cited

Deleuze, Gilles. *Crítica y clínica*. Trans. Thomas Kauf. Barcelona: Anagrama, 1997.

Doane, Mary Ann. "The Clinical Eye: Medical Discourses in the 'Woman's Film' of the 1940s." *The Female Body in Western Culture*. Ed. Susan S. Suleiman. Cambridge: Harvard UP, 1985. 152–74.

Cyrulnik, Boris. *La maravilla del dolor: El sentido de la resiliencia*. Trans. Gustavo González-Zafra. Barcelona: Granica, 1999.

Frank, Arthur W. *The Wounded Storyteller. Body, Illness, and Ethics*. Chicago & London: U of Chicago P, 1997.

Gadamer, Hans-Georg. *El estado oculto de la salud*. Trans. Nélida Machain. Barcelona: Gelisa, 1996.

Schopenhauer, Arthur. *Meditaciones sobre el dolor del mundo, el suicidio y la voluntad de vivir*. Trans. Carmen García Trevijano. Madrid: Tecnos, 1999.

I. Strategies of Medical Discourse

Pleasure, Pain and the Discourses of Industry: The Disabled Body as Cultural Object

Mark Mossman
Western Illinois University

My wife and I want to have a child. With my medical history, though, we recognize that the conception of that child may be difficult. I am disabled – a single-leg amputee – and I have end-stage renal disease. An impending transplant surgery hanging over our heads causes us to realize that we now need to plan, to begin to take measures to guarantee that we will be able to have a child at some point in the future.

So yesterday I began a process with an infertility clinic. I say 'process' because, though at this moment I do not know which direction exactly our activity will go here, I do know that it will involve stages and steps, and that right now we are still in the beginning or opening stage: we are trying to find out if I am, indeed, fertile, potent, able to produce an heir. Often in males prolonged kidney disease leads to a condition, called 'maturation arrest', where the man's body, despite having normal hormonal levels and thus the capacity to produce normal sperm, is unable to create anything other than spermatic 'germ cells', which have the potential to be full-grown sperm, but for whatever reason cannot quite complete their development. If I am at this stage of illness, then I am, technically, infertile, and we will just have to wait until after the transplant to address this new issue. On the other hand, if I do not have this condition – if my sperm are numerous and healthy – then we may now be able to cryo-preserve some of them in order to give us another option for conception after the transplant. More than anything, you see, is the consideration of the timing of it all: on the positive side, statistics show that, even if I now have 'maturation arrest' problems, sperm quality does often improve in males 9 to 12 months after the transplant; on the negative side, however, sometimes there are libido and resulting fertility problems with males after transplant surgery due to the immunosuppressant drugs.

One aspect in this early series of tests involves a basic analysis of my sperm, an assessment of its 'quality'. Yesterday morning, therefore, I went to the clinic for the first of several visits. After doing some paperwork and getting a few instructions from the nurse, I locked myself in a small, windowless room with a couch, a desk, a chair, and a small bathroom to the side, and proceeded to masturbate into a clear, latex condom. I had a number of material 'aids' to work with – magazines hidden in the desk, like 'Cheri', 'Barely Legal', 'Hustler', 'Penthouse', and 'Playboy' – and I had one hour to complete the job. I got into the room, sat down on the couch, decided I needed to use the bathroom, quickly got up and used the bathroom, sat back down on the couch, and tried to get 'comfortable'. After a few minutes, and after deciding that I did indeed need to open up the desk drawer and get out the pornography, I laughed quietly to myself: I saw the humor in all of this, the real pathos of producing semen for 'analyses'. I wondered out loud, 'Where were the candlelight and the soft music?' Initially, I was not really that nervous; I was just uncomfortable. I was becoming increasingly more so. As I thumbed through one of the magazines, again trying to become aroused, I felt the real strangeness of it all. Slowly, really to my surprise, I became deeply embarrassed, anxious, filled with worries and questions. Would it be hard to make eye-contact with the nurses when I left the room and went back out into the lab? Would they rate, for example, how much ejaculate I produced compared to other males my age? Would they note how much time I took to produce it? Should I go fast, then? Should I go slowly? And anyway, what would be the best, most appropriate way to get comfortable? Should I take off my shoes, and my socks, and my trousers? Should I sit down, or lie down, or stand up? How many people had used this couch before? And how often did they clean this room?

I felt the strangeness of the activity because, simply, it *was* strange: I was performing a historically deviant activity in a public, supposedly normalized situation; I was doing something with my body, in public, that our culture constructs and normalizes as a deeply private, personal activity. Though the door was closed and locked and privacy was, in other words, at least simulated, I was still, in a sense, out in the open, in the public's gaze. I was unsure of the rituals here, of what was appropriate and what was not. I did not want to do anything 'abnormal', and I knew that I did not know, in this circumstance, what was normal and what was not. I realize now, though, that that uncertainty is exactly what this experience and my past experiences of the medical industry are all about; that is why medicine is, to me, very powerful, very mystical in its control and dominance. When such a typically private, ritualized activity as sexual performance is suddenly governed by a larger industry, placed in a new set of discourses, actually managed and performed in an industry-space, a room in a medical clinic, the subject/patient suffers a tremendous loss of power in the dynamic of meaning. In that room medical science overtook my body, made my body its own, determined my body's performance and ability; in that room, masturbation was not a means of my own self-pleasure or gratification, but the requirement of the laboratory that was doing a standard 'semen analysis' test which, by the way, had a rather expensive price of $ 77. Sexual pleasure itself was in a significant way re-written by medicine, then, in that it was simply and cuttingly reduced to nothing more than behavior that would result in the production of the material to be analyzed, tested, reported on and profited from. My awkwardness was a symptom of a kind of somatic colonization, the deep penetration of exploitative discourses, the suddenly explicit dominance of my body by a larger 'industry'. The discourses and semantics of this industry expanded beyond the immediacy of the single moment. In larger terms, sitting in that room, trying to get aroused, I was suddenly aware that the eventual conception of my child, my offspring, my heir, would now, no matter what, be governed and perhaps even performed by the technology of the profit-driven, corporate-controlled, largely faceless medical industry.

As I have already hinted at above, and indeed have argued elsewhere,[1] I believe that in reality the patient's/disabled person's body has only two options when it finds itself in such hostile, uncomfortable, vaguely colonial situations: (1) the person can knowingly (and cunningly) play inside of post-modernity; can, in other words, 'sell out', 'let go', allow themselves to be taken by the circumstance, in this case a definable industry, and constructed as 'abnormal', 'ill', 'diseased', 'sick', 'pathological', as an industry-object; or (2) the person can resist, resist the post-modernity of the circumstance, and as a result become even stranger, more abnormal in his unwillingness to submit and give his individual body to the industry, a body which has been by now already designated, standardized and targeted by the industry.

This article concerns the hard social negotiation and real sense of post-modernity involved in following the first option. Sometimes, though, like yesterday as I left the clinic, I find myself articulating the emotions of the second option. I often want to resist or rebel, and in my illusionary, private, increasingly furious moments, I do. In such moments, like now, for example, right now as I am sitting here alone at my much-loved desk, in my quaint, small office, in the quiet basement of my rural home, empowered by my still-agile fingers deftly touching the keyboard in front of me, in these powerfully private moments I become a real voice in the wilderness, a wild prophet eating locusts and speaking fire, a lost fanatic screaming at the faceless demons that

1 See the following two articles: 'Visible Disability in the College Classroom.' *College English* 64 (July 2002): 645–59, and 'The One-Legged Wonder and Other Names.' *Post Identity* 3 (Winter 2002): 31–47.

haunt every step, a mad, madman whispering visions to the beautiful pictures and photographs hanging on the walls of his solitary cell. I become, more than anything, an angry man, standing single and firm in opposition to the great enemy of all that is 'natural' and 'organic' and 'good', the techno-medical industrial complex.

In these moments my rage boils into bitter constructions and re-tellings of my own history. I speak to myself in clear, basic terms. I tell myself, frantically striking the keys now, that I have been involved in a significant way with medical practice and medical doctors my entire life, that since I was just a few days old, for example, there has never been a day in my life where I have not taken a prescribed medication, something designed by the medical industry to manage some part of my body, to solve some problem suddenly articulated in my body and its systems. I tell myself that my somatic life has been dominated, controlled, and in a very real sense constructed by the United States medical industry. I whisper, quietly, to myself, that I am its product, and its child, and its heir; I articulate its deep, often hidden desires; I embody its troubled, darkly ambitious history and its glorious, triumphant understanding of its self.

And then I scream out that I despise and hate this industry because it is an industry that, to a large extent, aggressively makes meaning, possessively owns meaning, controls and disseminates meaning and wrecks those individuals who try to have some volition in the development of the meaning of their own lives. Medicine does not treat illness! It constructs reality itself in an attempt to structure and re-structure the 'ill' body! It is just an old-fashioned, Foucaldian power play, and they – the doctors, the nurses and the other industry workers – unconsciously control and construct it all, manage and run it all, while I sit, along with all of the other disabled, chronically ill patients, far outside of the discursive circles of authority and agency.

I sit at my desk, my hands now still before me, my body tensed and angered, for I can see, I can see vividly, that when you are chronically ill a clear pattern develops for your life where a doctor tells you how you feel, how you should feel, and often scolds you if you react inappropriately, or resist, or if you try to deviate from the way the doctor wants the pattern to go. My illness, my life, has been constructed, set up and planned out by someone other than myself, someone without a real face, someone wearing a white coat, reading a bunch of numbers on a chart, interpreting them without once really looking at me – which is not a 'medicalized' me, that is a set of numerical, chemical measurements, a group of highlighted proteins, creatine levels, and blood cell counts, but a 'me' or self who walks out of that office, out of that medical building, into the larger and much more significant worlds of family, career and community.

This anger, and this knowledge, translates, certainly, into my everyday behavior. But I am old now in my experience. And I am careful. I am under control. I use my anger. It is my gift, my right, my inheritance. I have seen and felt some things, and though I can still get bullied and intimidated, I do have a little bit of a swagger when I go in for my regular doctor's 'visit'. Of course I know that that swagger can be eliminated with one glance, one soft word from the doctor; all he has to do (and it is always a he) is read my chart and tell me of something, translate from the numbers there something obscure and dangerous, something I could never even envision as a possibility on my own. But still, often I at least put on a good show, maybe too much of a good show. Maybe I am getting too cocky. Last week, for example, when I went to the doctor I wanted to tell him – and, oh my God, I just about did – that he and his doctor friends are no different than the marginalized worker at McDonald's who serves me my Big Mac and a coke. They are not high and mighty. They are not Gods walking among mortal men. They are not above me or anyone else. They do not know as much about my body as I do. They are a service industry, and their purpose is simply to help me to get better – just like the fast food joint that serves me my food 'fast' and 'hot', my physician needs to diagnose and treat my illness 'accurately' and 'effectively'. Furthermore, I should be and, in fact, am the main and exclusive decision maker. Everything is my choice; they serve me. I pay their bills with my insurance; I am their customer. So, if I do not want to feel any pain or discomfort I should not have to feel any pain or discomfort. And further, if I do not want to go on dialysis, then I will not. If I do not want to start a new medication that I feel may be too debilitating, then I will not. If I do not want to do a surgical procedure that I find unnecessary, then I will not. If I just want to stay home, stay down in my own basement, down in my own office, then I will, and they cannot say or do anything to stop me.

But of course I know that this is never how it works. In my case, this open resistance (again the second option in my formulation) is not really open and is not, therefore, really resistance; it is just an elaborate fantasy. It is the boasting of a foolish coward who is right now safe in the maze of language, in the privacy of a discursive space he has created and maintained through 'private' writing that, at this point, no one else has even seen. This is my 'work'; this is my game; in a profound sense, I am both author and audience here. In reality, out there, outside of this office, outside of this work, doctors tell you (me) what to do. And you (me) do what they say, because you, as the patient, are supposed to do what they say, no questions asked, no resistance at all. Any anger you have is pointless, impotent, and often does nothing but harm to yourself; put simply, it is just foolishness and silliness to even really try to resist, to place your lone, solitary, ill body in opposition to, basically, an overwhelmingly immense industry that has the weight and wealth of the entire Western hemisphere behind it. How can anybody, really, resist such a thing? And why would anybody, really, resist, especially if you honestly, desperately want to live? When one places oneself in opposition, when one disagrees with the great physician, one makes oneself all the more strange and abnormal to that physician: the role of the patient is to obey and follow orders; Sander Gilman and many other researchers have proven, over the years, that patients who do not do this, who do not quickly and passively obey and follow the orders of the great doctor, are understood to be, simply, deviants. Again, with what is on the line in this relationship, why would the ill person want to risk clouding it with any kind of claim to power?

And indeed, in all honesty, despite the seemingly open, angry, and resistant thoughts above, I have always really wanted to do what my doctors have asked me to do. I always choose, as I have already documented, the first option: without hesitation, both metaphorically and physically, I sell out and let go of my body; I use my body, the different able and disabled constructions of it, to my advantage whenever I can, although I recognize that I cannot always control each construction, every formulation of my body. My only power play in this game is to let go and just play; play their games with my own interests secretly in mind. Indeed, in a sense, my own physical conditions are so complex and unusual that I am simply not able to make certain kinds of decisions on my own. My extreme, 'challenging',[2] body demands the extreme knowledge and skill of both the renal and urological specialist. In fact, I have always gone almost exclusively to specialists (right now, for example, I don't have a General Practitioner; I only work with the transplant team). And I try to trust them, to work with them. Again, I play their games, with my own interests in mind. I attempt to make them be what they want to be: true heroes, the great healers doing magic with their technological skill, the holy miracle workers on a noble mission to save lives, the architects of a transhistorical, transnational, transpolitical future, where death itself, that unnatural *struldburg* of little economic worth, will be thwarted step by step, cell by cell, disease by disease.

* * *

2 Yesterday the fertility expert described my 'case' as 'challenging'.

Perhaps at this point in my argument, it would be best to present some kind of researched evidence in order to support my position, to give critical context to the experience, thoughts and feelings I have outlined above. I have decided, however, to avoid the inclusion of research here in this essay. I think the citation of research would cloud the real heart of this project; this is a kind of autobiographical criticism, a kind of theoretical inquiry rooted completely in the context of my own experiences. I claim these experiences and I present them to you dear reader, without the encumbrance of academic research and the jargon associated with that kind of writing. I am now, legitimately, and briefly, out in the open, without those last, best defenses of the academy and the practices of scholarship to cloak, hide and protect me.

And, as is usual for anyone with a visible disability, being out in the 'open', being public, means being directly involved in and with paradox, complication and contradiction. My position here and in the larger project of my work as a whole is that, again, postmodern disability studies teaches us that, when one is rendered as 'abnormal', one sometimes must 'sell out', let their body be taken up and re-made by the 'normal' world around them, for often for the disabled, disfigured, ill body this movement, this strategic capitulation of the body, is the only way to survive the sociology around it; sometimes, in fact, as I have demonstrated, these painful moments of stereotype and exclusion can eventually lead to a deeper skill in the ability to define the meaning of one's experience and, arguably, one's 'self'. In postmodernity, enslavement to stereotype and freedom from it are often tangled up together;[3] the best strategy for the postmodern disabled body is to just glide, swim in and out of the different social constructions of abnormalcy, while at the same time trying hard to manage

3 Examples of this point can be gathered from current American television culture: it has been effectively argued that *Will and Grace* and *Queer Eye for the Straight Guy* are shows that both embody and dispel stereotypes of gay culture.

circumstances so that one is more volitional in one's behavior than not.

As I have already said, I recognize, though, that these strategies do not always work, and indeed this essay has already demonstrated how, in a certain circumstance, my body was overtaken, my volition thwarted by a larger discourse and industry; despite my sensitivity to issues concerning the body, and despite my ability to often avoid powerlessness and abnormalcy through deception and cloaking. At the infertility clinic yesterday my body, like many bodies systematically processed through the modern medical industry, was overridden and re-configured by the practice of a medical discourse, by the medical industry itself. Obviously, this type of powerlessness has occurred more than once in my life. The personal narrative at the start of this article dealt directly with an experience of 'pleasure' as it worked in a modern medical discourse and activity. I will now narrate a similar moment of 'pain'.

In 1997, when I was first diagnosed with end-stage renal failure, I was treated as a 'standard' body. Much of my medical history was, incredibly and embarrassingly, either lost or forgotten by myself (I was a child when most of the history's events took place), by my parents (they often buried facts as a way of coping with the intense pressure of having a sick child), and by the office of medical records at the hospital (and there is, in my opinion, no excuse here). During the early stages of the kidney transplant work-up, then, before my body was again discovered to be so completely non-standard, I often found myself in confusing, painful, difficult circumstances. One such circumstance happened the morning I was scheduled to do a number of basic 'work-up' tests.

I went to the lab that morning with determination. I was trying my best to be positive and focused; I was very unwilling at the time to be regarded as 'ill', and very suspicious of those who, in my mind, wanted to make me ill. I was younger, had had a remarkably good run of health, and was in the midst of both completing a dissertation on 19th century British literature and preparing an intensive search for the coming fall's academic job market. Needless to say, I was resistant, ambivalent, arrogant, confident, anxious and confused all at once, and on about three different levels of my existence: the development of my scholarship and thinking, my academic career, and now, suddenly, my basic health.

So I arrive at the lab very early in the morning, and at first it is okay. The techs are nice, and I do a simple ultra-sound, an EKG to test my heart, and a chest x-ray to test my lungs. Then I go back to the waiting area. I have one test left, a test about which I am very nervous. The test is called a cystotherogram. What happens in it is really quite simple: the technicians insert a dye into the bladder through a catheter and then, while the patient is lying on their back on the table, take an x-ray as h/she urinates the dye back out onto the table. The notion is to see if the dyed solution is urinated out of the bladder completely as it should be – sometimes with kidney disease patients, during urination some of the dye (and urine) is either retained or, and this is much worse, flushed back up into the kidney, which is a very specific kind of condition called 'reflux', and which of course could be very problematical for a transplanted organ and the transplant patient.

For a number of reasons, I was scared to death of catheterization. Among my physical anomalies is the fact that I have a somewhat disfigured penis (though it is not dramatic or clearly expressed). Put simply the urethra is not articulated in the normal place, but is instead slightly off-center, on the bottom tip of the penis, below where it should be.

My penis, then, presented, I thought with anxiety, a special problem. Most of all, though, I was not quite sure if the doctors were listening to my fears and worries: I felt that I was being rushed along, and I felt that they, the doctors, were unaware of what they were dealing with, that they were, essentially, making decisions in the dark; but, without even looking at my penis, and with only obscure, vague responses from me (responses again based on cloudy memory), they thought that the test should be 'standard', no special changes, no special pain killers.

I now lie on the large metal table in the x-ray room. The test is about to get underway. I wear only a blue buttoned down oxford and a pair of brown socks; over the shirt, I am covered by a white wrap-around, short-sleeved gown. My legs and my pelvic area are completely naked. I have a thin blue cotton blanket over me to keep me warm.

My prosthetic limb lies to the side. I feel very disabled without it. I feel vulnerable. But it is over there now, a few feet beyond my grasp. I don't want to get any of the dye on it, and I know it would probably be in the way when they put in the catheter.

I am exposed. My deepest secrets are there for public consumption – my scarred abdomen, my disfigured penis, my lack of a left limb. I am scared of the coming pain and mildly ashamed of my body. The pity card is there too. I see it in the nurses' and in the techs' faces. I can play it if I want to, but I am too tired, too nervous, too out in the open now. I close my eyes and try to let my mind spin easier. Really, all I want to do is to get through the exam. I tell myself to just let go of all this tension, worry and uncertainty, to just put my head down, and push through.

Finally, after about 40 minutes of waiting, another, different nurse comes in. She tells me that she is from the ER, and that she is there to do the catheter, while one of the techs will take the pictures.

I am unveiled. I ask the nurse, jokingly, not to hurt me. But I can see that she can see the fear in my face. And then, as I pull the blanket off me, and the gown all the way up, exposing myself completely, I can see the sudden, what would you call it, fear maybe? Curiosity? Uncertainty? Confusion? It is all there, one emotion after the next, quietly cloaked under the straining mask of professionalism as she closely examines my dorsal-holed penis looking for the right place to put in the catheter. With a little uncertainty, the nurse asks me if I have ever had this done before. My response is as it always is – 'drift'; 'glide'; 'sell out'. I don't want to cause any problems; I don't want to be any more abnormal than is already the case. I want to be agreeable, smooth, to say the right things and make the whole thing go along quickly and easily. I definitely do not want to show her, the nurse, how scared I really am. So I say, yes, that I think I probably had this test done a long time ago, when I was a child, but that I don't remember it clearly.

She tells me to relax, and then she inserts the tube.

White hot pain. I arch my back and groan. I did not want to make a sound; I just wanted to do it, get it over with. But the groan came out despite myself; my body responded outside of my own will and determination; my body experienced deep pain and automatically, amazingly and frighteningly responded to it.

She quickly draws the catheter back. Okay, she says, okay, let's try it again. She tries it again, and again burning pain. Sweat has now broken out on my forehead. I look down, and at the bottom of my torso I see my poor penis with a white tube sticking out of the bottom of it. I tell her, with control that amazes me really, that she needs to get it out, get the thing out.

She does, and contracts her brow nervously, confusedly, and asks me if I know whether or not I have had any strictures. I say no, not sure what 'strictures' are, but instinctively I know what she means.

I felt an obstruction, she then says. You think you may have some scar tissue?

I shrug and stare at the ceiling. I do not know. I am ignorant of my body. I only know that it hurt terribly a moment ago, that it still stings a little now, and that I want to reach down and hold on to my penis, to try to stop the stinging pain, but that I should not do that, that I should keep my hands to my side and let the nurses do their job. I now know that, in other words, I am tremendously uncertain about everything. I am trying to maintain my composure, to retain some control over my surroundings. But I now have this need to avoid eye-contact; I desperately want this test to be over; and I do not want to do anything silly, or foolish. I am realizing that I have already done so, though. This is non-standard; this is all strange and abnormal.

The nurse calls for a smaller catheter. Other nurses come in. They hover over me, as the ER nurse tries the new one. Same result. It gets stuck right at the top of my penis, right when it is about an inch in. And it hurts – a bald, naked pain – and I groan with the pain, my body flinching and twisting with the pain, my hands clenching the sides of the cold, metal table, the growing number of nurses around me holding down my arms and shoulders, giving me strange, bizarre words of encouragement like, you're doing great, Mark, and, you can do it, c'mon Mark, you can do this.

I now know that at that particular spot my urethra narrows to a fine point, and that, indeed, the entire urethra is non-standard, unusually shaped, 'friable' and 'torturous' – to use the doctor's terms – a looping, twisting, turning thing that is like a roller coaster and is almost impossible to navigate, and certainly impossible to do so while I am conscious and able to feel pain. I now know that in order to get the catheter in, the urologists must first knock me out, and then use a 'French Scope' and a steel rod that allows them to carefully push the tubing through the twisting maze that is my urethra to the bladder. At the time, of course, I was not sure what was going on. I only knew that I was slowly losing control of my body and of the entire situation spinning around my body. I was afraid, in pain, and unable to control anything around me or, seemingly, within my own body.

After some discussion, and a call for an urologist, the nurses discuss the possibility of trying another catheter, the smallest one they have, one that is a child's size. It flashes through my mind that this might be demeaning – using a child-sized catheter on a 27 year-old man, but I don't care. Again, I just want it over with, and I do not want to be silly or foolish or a coward.

After about 20 minutes, the urologist is still not there, so they decide, with my approval, to try the child's one anyway. I get ready, shut my eyes, get simultaneously tensed, anticipating pain, and relaxed, in order to minimize pain. The nurse inserts the tiny catheter and at first it is okay, tolerable. And then it hurts, a hard, penetrating pain, a pain that makes my leg and my amputated stump kick up, involuntarily. Despite my effort to stay calm and quiet, to just take it, I again grunt and groan with the sharp pain, my body, literally, jerking and twisting back in its response.

At this point, the nurse quickly pulls the catheter back out, and we all decide, much to everyone's relief, to quit now and just do this test on another day with the urologist from the transplant team. Without any more real communication, everyone leaves the room, and I slowly, tenderly, get up, put on my prosthetic limb and my clothes, walk out of the hospital into daylight and to my parked car, and drive home, shaken and terribly embarrassed. I had a tremendous, burning sensation every time I urinated for about a week.

* * *

It took me a long time to write about the painful experience above. It is still close; I am still in danger, I think, of having experiences like the one above. Such is life: indeed, my point is now to demonstrate, in this final section of this paper, how it is a particular kind of life, a specific type of knowledge or perspective.

I believe that, historically, the cultural marginalization grounded in disability or physical abnormalcy leads, historically, to certain kinds of rhetorical strategies (i.e., compulsive autobiography) and a resulting dynamic of cultural structures or configurations (i.e., for the disabled/physically abnormal person the sense of an alien status and an equally strong desire to cloak oneself in normalcy). Postmodern disability studies have provided a new perspective or critical paradigm, however, through which one can now seriously re-evaluate the experiences of the disabled body. More than anything, that perspective demonstrates how normalcy works, how it is sometimes challenged and undermined by visibly abnormal bodies, and how, unfortunately, when one is visibly abnormal one must still sometimes 'glide', 'sell out', 'do what is necessary', even when doing so results in negative stereotype, discrimination or exploitation. I believe further that the perspective of the new disability studies also demonstrates cultural connection, a definite solidarity between those individuals or groups that are often the objects of industry discourses and thus the victims of harsh, mostly economic exploitation. In this sense, I believe that there is always a possibility of empowerment: there is always a door to go through, an escape hatch to find, a different set of discourses with which one can align one's self and experiences.

To a point, this connection is discovered through a simple analysis of discourse and discursive practice. For example, the basic differences of terminology in describing one of my own medical conditions illustrate this distinction in discursive power and demonstrates the way that a cultural industry reaches out and takes control of its targeted object, in this case my own ill, visibly disabled body. Put simply, often my experience is reworked through medical perspective, literally re-made and given a different meaning, through the different words used by the powerful physician. So, tomorrow or next week or next month I'll go to my doctor and tell him, 'I am having pissing problems today'; the doctor will say, 'You are experiencing urinary retention'. I'll say, 'Yes, the piss feels like it's getting stuck right in the middle of my prick, like I can just not quite get it out of me'. The doctor will then reply, 'Though it is unlikely, there may be an obstruction or stricture in the urethra'. I'll say, 'I'm having problems with dripping as well; I often feel like I'm never done, and that I could just stand or sit there for hours letting the piss slowly drip out of me'. The doctor will tell me, 'You are experiencing periods of incontinence'. I'll say, 'Right. But I was shut down totally for about five hours last night. Not even a drop came out. It was awful and uncomfortable and frightening. I was unsure of what I should do'. The doctor will say, knowingly, 'You most likely experienced a pelvic floor spasm'. I'll then say, 'Okay. Got it. Sometimes, though, I feel so swelled up it is like I will burst. I feel it when I stand up, or walk and I can only get comfortable when I am sitting down'. The doctor will say, politely, 'You are having difficulty voiding the bladder'. I'll say, 'Yes. Right again. I piss at least every hour, and sometimes more, sometimes every 30 minutes, or, when I am having pissing problems, every 20 minutes. I always have to go, and when I am going well I just piss gallons'. The doctor will say, 'You are experiencing a sense of urgency'. I'll say, finally, 'Help me, man; I hate this; this is not right; this is seriously changing the way I go about my life'. The doctor will say, finally, 'It appears to be a functional problem, for which there is no solution'.

What occurs in these kinds of conversations, where the physician essentially re-writes the condition described by the patient, re-states it in different terms for the patient, ultimately provides some final end-statement or resolution for the patient, is a simple power play: by re-making the condition, re-naming it in a medicalized discourse, the doctor takes a kind of ownership of the condition, and of the body that is experiencing the condition; the doctor takes the body of the patient from the patient. Further, the doctor becomes the source of a cure, is the only one who can make the body well. It is understood that if the doctor cannot make the patient well again, no one and no thing can. In every possible way, then, the doctor becomes the religious – in the full sense of that term – master of the whole terrible, awful, pathetic situation: you learn to speak, to mimic the doctor's holy words; you let the omnipotent doctor define what you experience and explain to you what that experience means; you pray that the blessed doctor will make your sinful body well again, to stop the trouble that has fallen upon your suddenly very corruptible body.

But there is more going on here; post-modernity has altered, ever so slightly, the relationship between the physician and the patient. Again, I believe critically that, like feminist or ethnicity studies, the analysis of disability and the perspective of the new disability studies, stretches into a larger reading of Western cultural practice in general. Disability study is, in the end, an analysis of power, of relationships and of the workings of culture. What the new disability studies can do, as an agent of cultural studies, is make larger connections, build up points of practical, real solidarity.

Based on what I have gathered from my own experience, for example, I assert that just as the porn star, the industry-girl, in a hard-core pornographic film lets her body get degraded on film in awful positions by awful people, in tabooed places that causes both pleasure and pain, often 'the patient', in his day-to-day life, in order to survive, must let himself be degraded by a medical industry that is looking only to exploit the body, to place it in various odd, strange circumstances, for profit and, indirectly, for a level of self-gratification. The disabled person, likewise, is on the same track, confronts the same kinds of cultural structures of exploitation and stereotype. In this context, and in personal terms, my life as a chronically ill, visibly disabled person has been equivalent to a cheesy, sleazy, XXX porn flick, where my body has had one medical encounter after the next, one exploitative experience after another. I am not the medical industry's child and heir; I am one of its pornographic stars.

What I am saying here is that my body, the temple in which I exist, the holy place housing my soul, is simply an industrial object, and is much akin to a pornographic body, or any other body rendered as abnormal by the tyranny of normalcy and exploited by a cultural industry as such. My very first experience with pornography illustrates this connection, this link through the discourses of industry.

My first serious, memorable encounter with pornography was when I was 12 years old. The routine was pretty simple: every Friday I'd get home from school, watch television until my parents got home, do the chores they required me to do (like gathering up my dirty clothes for the week, or helping my father take out the garbage), take a quick shower, eat supper, and then meet my best friend Darrin walking down Liberty Street. On most nights, depending on the time of year of course, we would then either go to the high school football game (or basketball game or baseball game), meeting other friends there, or we would go to 'the show', which meant that we would go to an old movie house in the center of town and pay $ 2.00 to see pretty much any movie we wanted, no matter what it was rated. After the show or the game, and no matter what the weather was, we would all, a group of usually four or five adolescent males, walk the long two mile stretch out to the edge of town where the new pizza places and arcades were.

On the way to the pizza place, from which I would walk home, sometimes by myself and often very late at night, there were a number of interesting sites for young, trouble-seeking adolescent males. There was a car dealership owned by my best friend's hated ex-stepfather where we could key cars; there was an old salvation army store where we could loiter and talk and smoke underneath an awning; there was a gas station where we could steal cigars and packs of gum; there was a fast food place where we could get sodas for free from one of my friends' older brothers; there was a dark alley where older kids took their dates and made out. By far the most important place we discovered, though, was an older garage, through which we could see a pin-up of a half-naked woman.

We could see this picture through a dusty window at the back of the building. I am not sure why we even went back there; I think we were looking for a short-cut to the strip mall, which was again our ultimate destination. But, when we were back there one of us, and I don't remember who, looked into the window and spotted the picture. It was amazing, great luck. A street light shone through the window and, though the rest of the room was obscure (it was probably the back office of the owner of the garage) and though I never once saw the picture in daylight, I remember that pin-up well; the woman was half-naked, and, to my profound fascination, it was the bottom half that was naked; she was young, dark-haired, and had very white skin and dark, shining eyes; she wore a pinkish-white sweater and a pair of white bobbed socks; she sat, on what appeared to be a group of white, fuzzy pillows, up-close to the camera, leaning back, staring directly into it, smiling, with her legs opened before you, so that you could see everything – her flat belly, her knees, the backs of her thighs, and her vagina, and the thick curls of silky black hair above and around it.

This photo was discovered one night, and we all, each one of us, took turns looking at it every Friday night for the rest of that school year.

I now realize that when I gazed at this photo, with my adolescent, male friends behind me, pushing at me to get their turn, I experienced a complicated complex of identity-building structures. I was disfigured, disabled, a deviant body; I was surrounded, literally, by a group of normalized, heterosexual male bodies; I was gazing at a sexualized, objectified representation of the female body. Importantly, I did not feel uncomfortable; I wanted to look; indeed, the real tension came in trying to discipline myself not to look too much, to be in control, to look just as much as everyone else: I did not want to be a pervert, to be abnormal, even though I knew that, if I was on my own, I would gaze at the body for a much longer stretch of time, that in fact I was deeply fascinated (not only sexually) by the representation. I struggled with the complexity of it all; I even remember telling myself that it was normal to want to look at the picture: at 12 I was Catholic, very religious, and so I simultaneously felt the impinging guilt of looking at the picture while I deeply longed to gaze at that sinful, tabooed picture.

I now know this: I was, in a sense, identifying with that picture, with that denigrated body. At the exact same time, I experienced a profound objectification and identification or alignment with that representation. My body, like the porn-industry body, is both normalized and abnormalized in cultural practice. Think about it: the porn-industry body is a body that is obscene, that is re-made in its performance, that is often 'enhanced', shaved, oiled, that is the location of both pleasure and disgust, that is represented as being natural and normal and filthy and abnormal all at once, at the exact same time. This kind of massive contradiction is comfortable to me, has always been comfortable to me, and I suspect it is comfortable for all industry-objects, no matter what the discourse industry may be.

In simple terms, then, porn defined the woman's body I was looking at: an industry placed it in a certain pose, represented it in a certain medium, distributed the representation of it throughout culture for a certain profit, made that woman's body mean something, something obscene, something sexualized. The woman's body was taken by an industry, made into an object of the industry. The terms of the larger industry came to define what her body meant, how it was presented to me.

At 12 I understood how industry-objects exist, what life meant, and I could easily read the body as such, and therefore I could also read a solidarity into the dynamic; I could and did identify on some level with the representation. The disabled body, my body, had the same characteristics of existence.

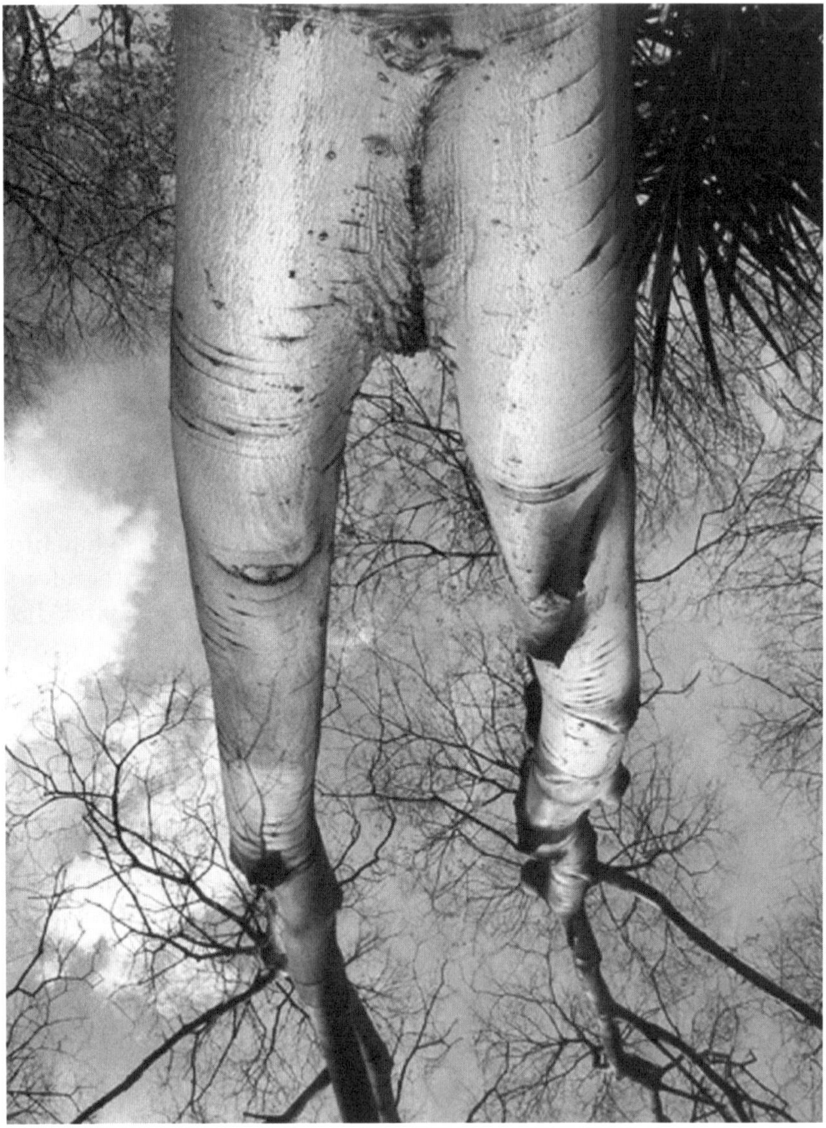

Rossana Zaera. "Heridas, cicatrices y otras condecorationes" (Wounds, Scars, and other Condecorations)

Pain as Expression: The Case of Hysteria

Ángel Cagigas
University of Jaén

Hysteria is an illness as old as human beings, the beauty of whose history is impossible to renounce. Authors in Antiquity already knew of it, the Egyptians diagnosed and cured it, but it was Hypocrates who after having absorbed their knowledge baptised it under the name of hysteria, not out of originality but out of precision because 'hystera' in Greek means uterus. The name thus refers to its cause, and is related to the displacements of the womb in a state of starvation. This argument was taken up by Plato in *Timaeus*, where he claimed that it is only when the uterus, eager for breeding, has not been fertilised for a long period that it wanders through the body and obstructs air canals, preventing breathing and unleashing various diseases (par. 91c).

From that period onwards, hysteria has not ceased to come up in Celsus's and Areteus de Capadocia's writings. It became manifest in Asclepios's temples and it was observed in medieval exorcisms. In each historical moment it has appeared through peculiar phenomena since one of its most prominent features is mimesis, i.e., its adaptation to the habits, behaviours, modes of thought and worries of a certain epoch. Seemingly, hysteria reacts to environmental demands, so that when the latter changes so does the form hysteria adopts. But there is a moment in history when hysteria reaches the height of its fame. In the second half of the twentieth century Jean Martin Charcot, probably one of the most distinguished inventors of modern neurology, turns hysteria into one of his major accomplishments.

After analysing a great number of pathological phenomena – i.e., chronic rheumatism, gout, ataxia, multiple sclerosis, aphasia,

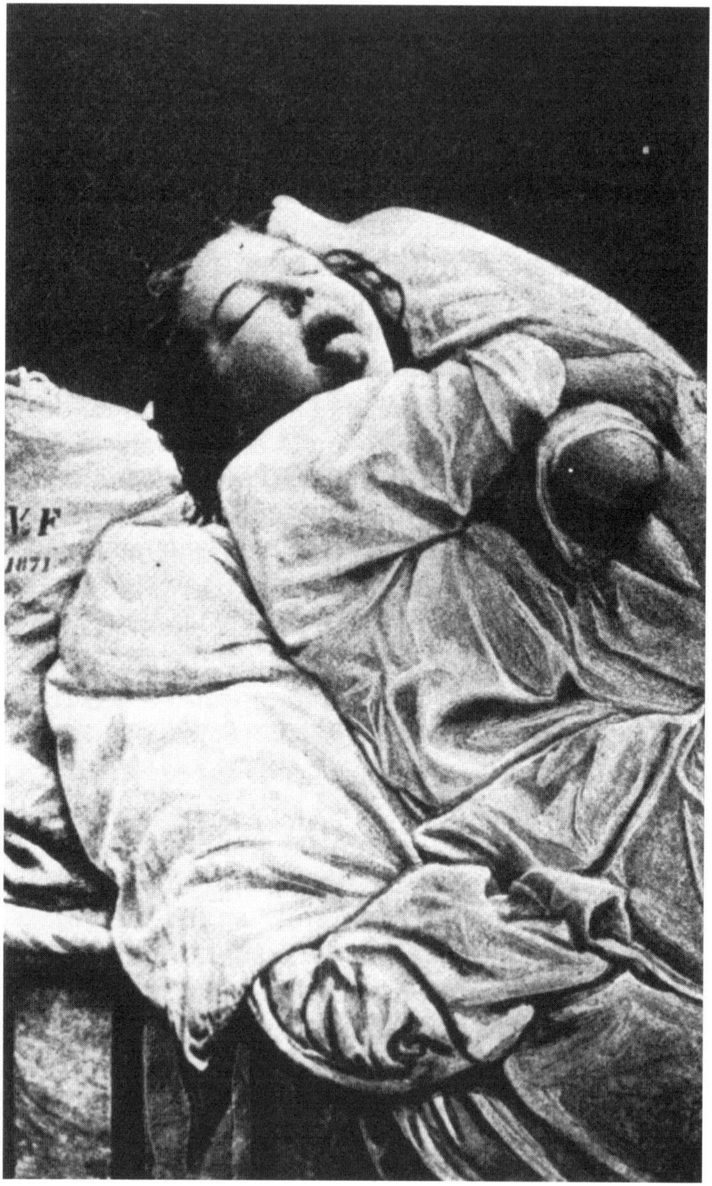

Epileptic Crisis. *Iconographie photographique de la Salpêtrière*, 1878.

brain haemorrhage, and amyotrophic lateral sclerosis –, from 1865 onwards Charcot devotes his time to hysteria. By then the status of hysteria as an illness was doubtful because a majority of doctors understood it as a fraud, a fictitious disease made up by young women wanting to avoid responsibilities. Charcot, however, believed that it was a real disease that attacked not just women but also men and children, and worked to find its cause, its symptoms, and a successful course of action.

From the beginning Charcot fights the idea of hysteria as a protean disease that escapes definition, as Briquet vehemently argues (5). Intent on classifying symptoms and causes, Charcot differentiates local signs – like anaesthesias, paralysis and contractures – from general indications, such as convulsions, fainting fits, hallucinations and deliria. However, behind the apparent diversity of its symptoms that mutate incessantly, Charcot underscores mimesis, i.e., the patients' tendency to imitate the symptoms they see in other patients, mainly epilepsy (*démoniaques* 91–103; *Leçons du mardi 1887–88*: 173–79, 101–2). As to its cause, at first he claims it is organic, resulting from a brain lesion caused by a degeneration of a congenitally weak nervous system. But, however much he strove to isolate this cerebral wound he was not able to locate it. So, in 1885 he elaborates a theory of trauma according to which hysteria – invisible, evanescent and dynamic – is produced by a brain dysfunction in individuals genetically predisposed to contract it. In them hysteria is unchained via various factors, such as accidents, fears, certain religious practices, typhus, diabetes, syphilis, tiredness, alcoholism, intellectual exhaustion, masturbation, smoking, continence or venereal excesses. Profession and race also weigh upon its appearance (*Clinique* 389). Charcot then traces the course of hysteria in four stages: epileptic, illogical, passionate and terminal (*démoniaques* 94–103). Often, however, the epileptic attack is preceded by a special feeling, 'the hysterical aura' (*démoniaques* 92–4), that announces the coming of the crisis through hallucinations, sensitivity disorders, and various organic disturbances. It is at this moment that Charcot takes pictures of his patients so as to use them later for research.

After the 'hysterical aura', epilepsy appears, so-called because it culminates in an epileptic crisis. The patient goes through three phases: Tonic – whose beginning is signalled by a cry followed by convulsions; clonal – characterised by spasms and violent contractures, and terminal or relaxing during which the body falls into a light sleep. The terminal phase is, in turn, followed by a stage of illogical postures: the patient's body twists up in the most implausible positions, as if it were possessed. Eventually, during the third stage the patient tries to express through different physical poses various emotions and feelings, be they aggressive, loving, saddening, or religious (*démoniaques* 102). One of the most prominent features of hysteria, theatricality, is made manifest at this time. All of this is documented by Charcot through hundreds of photographs that despite their beauty minutely convey the tragedy and pain of hysterics.

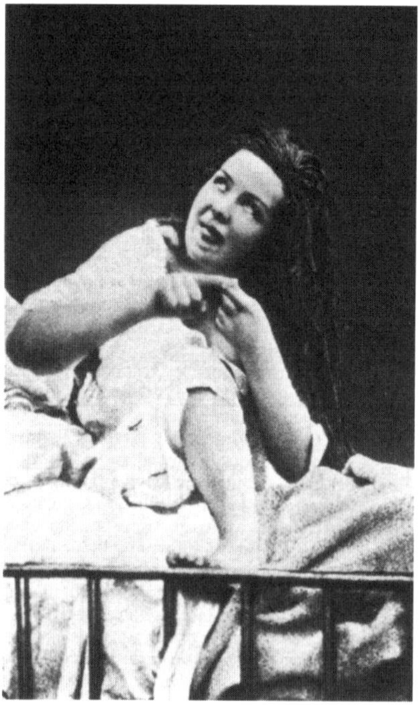

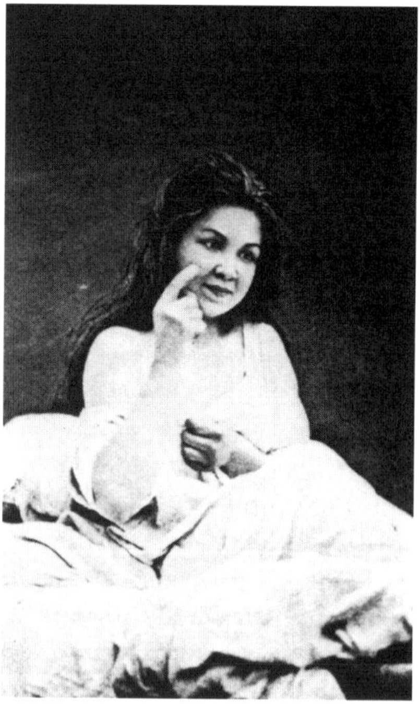

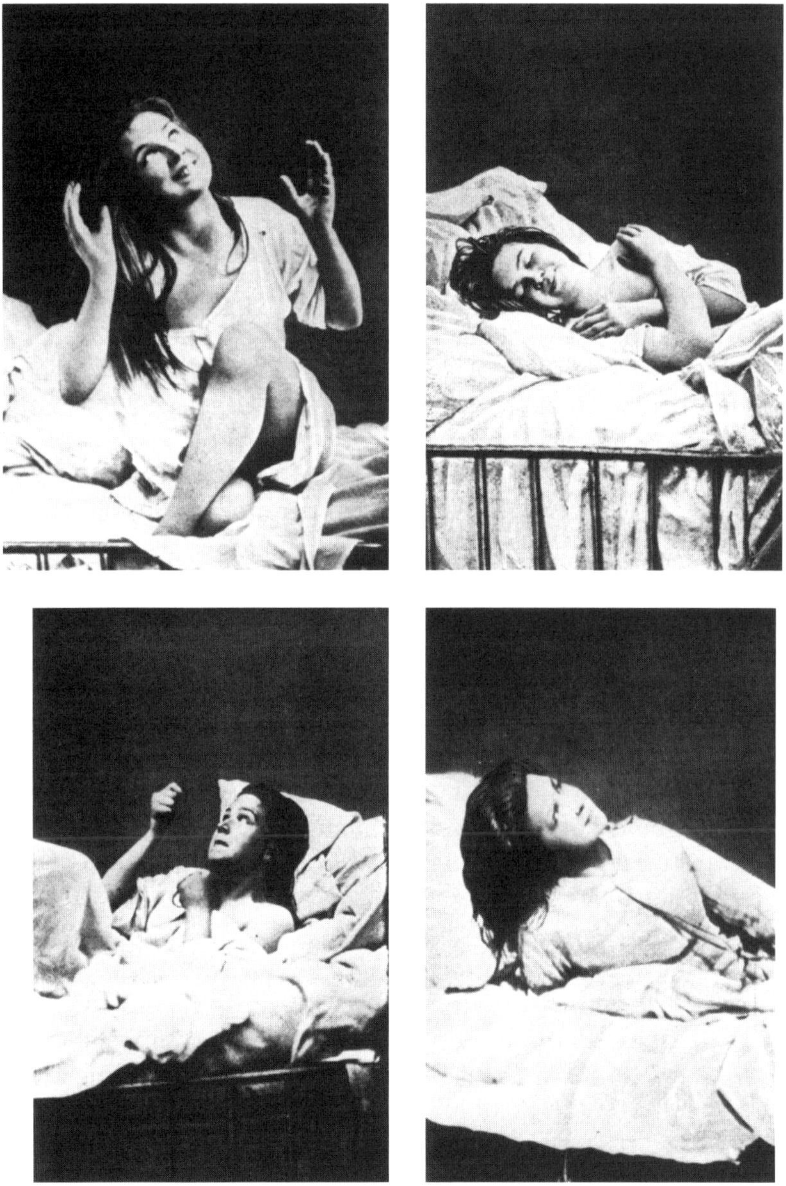

Passionate postures. *Iconographie photographique de la Salpêtrière,* 1878.

Throughout the terminal stage emotions are no longer performed. Patients partially recover their consciousness but instead develop motion problems. Cramps that may last minutes, hours, or even days, teary cries of pain from the many women interned at La Salpêtrière. In sum, the total duration of the hysterical attack is approximately 15 minutes, but it can repeat itself in a series of 10 or 20 attacks, occasionally reaching 200. It might also happen that one or several of these stages are missed, giving way to four different forms of frustrated crises, depending on the stage the patient should theoretically be going through.

A typical case is that of Rosalie Leroux, an hysterical woman who suffers all four stages and hundreds of attacks. She also presents stigmas, adopts the crucifixion poses of old demonic possessions, and confesses to having been in Heaven with Christ, the Virgin Mary and all the Saints. Hers is a story common among the patients at la Salpêtrière. She was abandoned as a child and was constantly abused by her wet-nurses. At 11 she was attacked by a dog and from then onwards she started to suffer convulsions with loss of consciousness. Years later she sees the dead body of a woman murdered at the hands of her husband who is then arrested. The scene exacerbates her nerves. At 19 she is the victim of a criminal who haunts her down in the woods. This episode paralyses the right side of her body. When she is 23, and after having suffered several crises of such violence that five or six people are required to hold her down, she is admitted to la Salpêtrière, where she is to remain for 40 years (*Leçons sur les maladies 1889*: 18).

Another typical example is that of Genevieve, abandoned as a child in Loudun, a town renowned for its 18th century witch processes. Apart from presenting stigmas, she succumbs to erotic frenzies, fantasies of a sexual nature, expressions of extreme lewdness and relives with great emotional intensity certain traumatic events in her past. All of which suggests, in Charcot's view, the underlying presence of emotional and passionate elements under hysteria (*Leçons sur les maladies 1872*: 300).

Once the pattern of the hysterical attack is structured, Charcot turns to its causes. In this matter he resorts to Reynolds' work on paralysis and movement disorders, to which he continually refers as the basis for his theory on the psychogenesis of hysteria. Reynolds' work is preceded by Brodie's and R.B. Carter's, where the temperamental basis of hysteria, its sexual aetiology – which often evolves into unsatisfied desire –, and the repression caused by social obligations, are established. They also typify diverse clinical frames and devise a treatment based on isolation, which will be often used by Charcot. The latter will eventually claim that hysteria is in truth an imaginary illness, not because it is not real but because, as Reynolds argued, and Paracelsus did before him, it depends on the images unconsciously created after a trauma. These images are transformed into acts by patients.

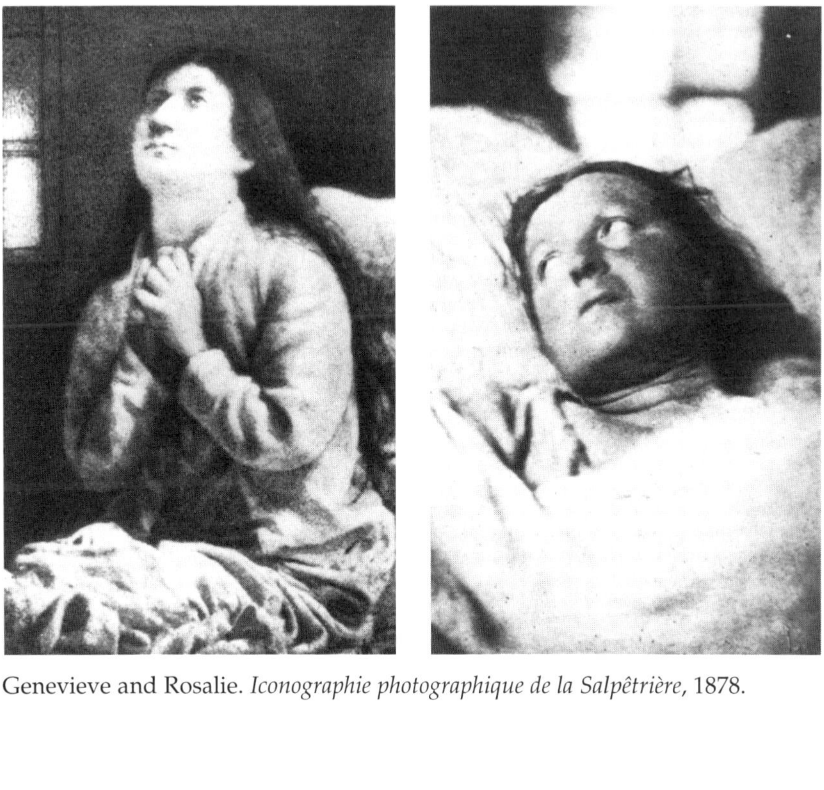

Genevieve and Rosalie. *Iconographie photographique de la Salpêtrière*, 1878.

In light of this argument Charcot becomes the target of fierce criticisms, the most important of which claims that he does not cure hysteria at la Salpêtrière, often called the 'city of pain', but rather cultivates it, as if he himself would be able to create it with the power of his will and the force of his imagination. He always responds to critique with sarcasm and a certain dose of humour:

> Il semble que l'hystéro-épilepsie n'existe qu'en France et je pourrais dire et on l'a dit quelquefois, qu'à la Salpêtrière, comme si je l'avais forgée par la puissance de ma volonté. Ce serait chose vraiment marveilleuse que je puisse ainsi créer des maladies, au gré de mon caprice et de ma fantaisie. Mais à la vérité, je ne suis absolument là que le photographe, j'inscris ce que je vois et il m'est trop facile de montrer que ce n'est pas à la Salpêtrière seulement que ces choses-là se passent. (*Leçons du mardi 1887–88*: 178)

It would be marvellous to make up diseases! However, hysteroepilepsy does not only exist in France, and, furthermore, a doctor is unable to make up a disease out of fantasy. Charcot was merely a photographer who recorded what he saw.

The plastic character of hysteria captivates many authors in the 19th century, the century of hysteria. Certainly, and outside the realm of medical practice, the word was already common before Charcot made it fashionable to refer to the vague desires of adolescents, the boredom of thirty year-old women, and the privations of middle-aged females who looked into the future turning their heads back, as Sarcey ingeniously notes in *Le mot et la chose:*

> Nous voyons déjà poindre un terme dont la fortune a été singulièrement rapide. Il est sorti des livres de médicine, et convient tout à fait à un siècle matérialiste qui ne voit dans l'homme qu'un sujet d'études physiologiques. C'est le mot 'hystérique'. On trouve aujourd'hui de l'hystérie partout. Ces troubles delicieux d'une jeune fille que ne forme que des désirs vagues et pleure sans savoir pourquoi: hystérie. Ces langueurs de la femme de trente ans qui s'ennuie et qui rêve: hystérie. Les aspirations tumultueuses de la femme de quarante ans qui s'élance dans l'avenir en retournant la tête: hystérie. Nos docteurs ont peuplé le monde d'hystériques. Ce mot n'est point agréable, il porte avec lui je ne sais quel parfum d'hôpital. Il

> est pourtant le bienvenu. Il se dégage peu à peu de ce cortège d'idées médicales dont il était entouré à sa naissance. Il finira par prendre une tournure tout à fait mondaine. (261)

Sometime after 1863, Maupassant, assiduous witness to Charcot's experiments, mocks the omnipresent diagnosis of hysteria, used to refer both to the Parisian commune and to the acquittal of Gabrielle Fénayrou, after being accused of complicity in the murder of her husband:

> Hystérique, madame, voilà le grand mot du jour. Êtes-vous amoureuse?, vous êtes une hystérique. Êtes-vous indifférente aux passions qui remuent vos semblables?, vous êtes une hystérique, mais une hystérique chaste. Trompez-vous votre mari?, vous êtes une hystérique, mais une hystérique sensuelle. Vous volez des coupons de soie dans un magasin?, hystérique. Vous mentez à tout propos?, hystérique! (Le mensonge est même le signe caractéristique de l'hystérie). Vous êtes gourmande?, hystérique! Vous êtes nerveuse?, hystérique! Vous êtes ceci, vous êtes cela, vous êtes en fin ce que sont toutes les femmes depuis le commencement du monde? Hystérique!, hystérique!, vous dis-je. Nous sommes tous des hystériques depuis que le docteur Charcot, ce grand prêtre de l'hystérie, cet éleveur d'hystériques en chambre, entretient à grand frais dans son établissement modèle de la Salpêtrière un peuple de femmes nerveuses auxquelles il inocule la folie, et dont il fait, en peu de temps, des démoniaques. Il faut être vraiment bien ordinaire, bien commun, bien raisonnable, pour qu'on ne vous classe point aujourd'hui parmi les hystériques. Les académiciens ne le sont pas, les sénateurs non plus. Tous les grands hommes le furent. (112)

Certainly, the word soon exceeds its etymology and with time loses its meaning. Maupassant, however, did not take into account that all the discoveries made by Charcot would not have been possible without a previous culture medium. It was precisely this atmosphere that allowed Flaubert to create Emma Bovary, fixating thus on a specimen that startled his contemporaries because of the medical precision of his style and descriptions. Just two years after the publication of Flaubert's masterpiece, Briquet describes in his famous *Traité clinique et thérapeutique de l'hystérie* the type of the hysterical woman. Some time later in *Le spleen de Paris*, Baudelaire paints Mademoiselle Bistouri (206–8) with a range of colours that coincides with the colours preferred and used by Charcot's patients, who sooner or later become models for many fictional heroines who end up enamoured of their Parisian doctors. Most famous are *Les amours d'un interne* (1881) by Jules Claretie, and *Germinie Lacerteux* (1875) by the Grancourt brothers, both the latter were intimate friends of Charcot. Their female protagonist is an adolescent who, after having been raped, works as a servant to courtesans who imbue her with a morbid affection for novels. In love with her confessor, Germinie, a drunkard, a sex addict, forever suffering and in search of pain, refers us to a real case, the double life of the Goncourts' maid, who, in her turn, also duplicates the life of the women who arrive at la Salpêtrière, targets of Charcot's and Bourneville's photographic lens. In fact, Charcot uses both reality and fiction as sources of inspiration. And, interestingly enough, writers attend his classes to take notes and highlight the verisimilitude of their works.

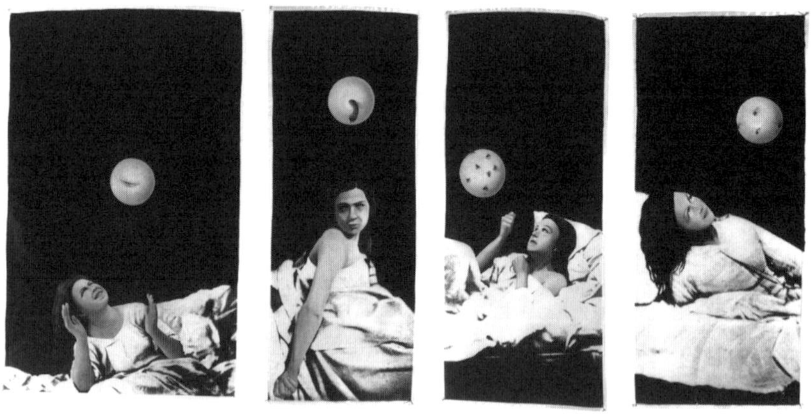

Marina Nuñez. *Locura (Madness)*, 1997.

The hysterical atmosphere not only affects the literary production in the epoch. Many of these writers also claim to be hysterical, as Charcot himself did in jest. In fact, there is a whole aesthetic movement that cannibalises Romanticism and converts illness into a metaphor for creativity, because it is only the presence of the other that paves the way to aesthetic creation. Baudelaire admits in 'Mon coeur mis à nu' to having cultivated his hysteria with both pleasure and horror:

> Au moral comme au physique, j'ai toujours eu la sensation du gouffre, non seulement du gouffre du sommeil, mais du gouffre de l'action, du rêve, du souvenir, du désir, du regret, du remords, du beau, etc. J'ai cultivé mon hystérie avec jouissance et terreur. (401)

Likewise, in *Le spleen de Paris* he describes the poet as a man given to contemplation, inactivity, dreaming and excess, driven by malicious devils who install themselves in his body and force him to perform their absurd desires: 'J'ai été plus d'une fois victime de ces crises et de ces élans, qui nous autorisent à croire que des démons malicieux se glissent en nous et nous font accomplir, a notre insu, leurs plus absurdes volontés' (167). But however painful eternal damnation might look, it eventually compensates the artist on allowing him to find just a second of infinite pleasure.

Saint-Beuve, a doctor himself, assumes a diagnosis of 'moral hysteria', and admits to being affected by a grief that still many consider exclusive to women. Whereas melancholy is expressed in Romantic poetry under the form of effusions and lyrical despair, soon it finds new style, as Barrès explains:

> Toi qui as abandonné le bohémianisme d'esprit, la libre fantaisie des nerfs pour devenir raisonnable, tu étais né cependant comme je suis né pour n'aimer que la grâce passagère de la vie et les désarrois des puissances de l'âme. Ta jeune hystérie se plaisait dans la souffrance. (117)

But maybe Flaubert is the first, the most typical, and the most excessive example that we remember. He diagnoses himself hysterical, in fact, he claims to be an hysterical woman. In one of his letters to George Sand – dated 12 January 1867, in which he comments on the solitude in which he lives and works at Croisset –, he maintains that men can be as hysterical as women, and he further declares that this torture is the only experience worthy of being lived, thus paring, as Baudelaire did, pain and pleasure:

> La sensibilité s'exalte démesurément dans un pareil milieu. J'ai des battements de coeur pour rien (chose comprensible, du reste, dans un vieil hystérique comme moi). Car je maintiens que les hommes sont hystériques comme les femmes et que j'en suis un. Quand j'ai fait *Salammbô*, j'ai lu sur cette matière-là 'les meilleurs auteurs' et j'ai reconnu tous mes symptômes. J'ai la boule et le clou à l'occiput: tout cela résulte de nos jolies occupations. Voilà ce que c'est que de se tourmenter l'âme et le corps. Mais si ce tourment-là est la seule chose propre qu'il y ait ici bas...

In his next letter on 15 January 1867, he introduces the theme of the artist's bisexuality on discussing his love for Severino. Why would such a disease need a sex? Sand does not remain silent:

> Qu'est-ce au fond que d'être hystérique? Je l'ai peut-être été aussi, je le suis peut-être, mais je n'en sais rien, n'ayant jamais approfondi la chose et en ayant ouï parler sans étudier. N'est-ce pas un malaise, une angoisse causée par le désir d'un impossible *quelconque*? En ce cas, nous en sommes tous atteints, de ce mal étrange, quand nous avons de l'imagination; et pourquoi une telle maladie aurait-elle un sexe?

In fact, Baudelaire turns Emma into Flaubert's double, a game Flaubert indeed celebrates claiming that he himself is Madame Bovary. Baudelaire will look deeply into this matter considering the possibility of an hysterical art:

> L'hystérie! Pourquoi ce mystère physiologique ne ferait-il pas le fond et le tuf d'une oeuvre littéraire, ce mystère que l'École de Médicine n'a pas encore résolu, et qui, s'exprimant dans les femmes par la sensation d'une boule ascendante et asphyxiante (je ne parle que du symptôme principal), se traduit chez les hommes nerveux par toutes les impuissances et aussi par l'aptitude à tous les excès? (481)

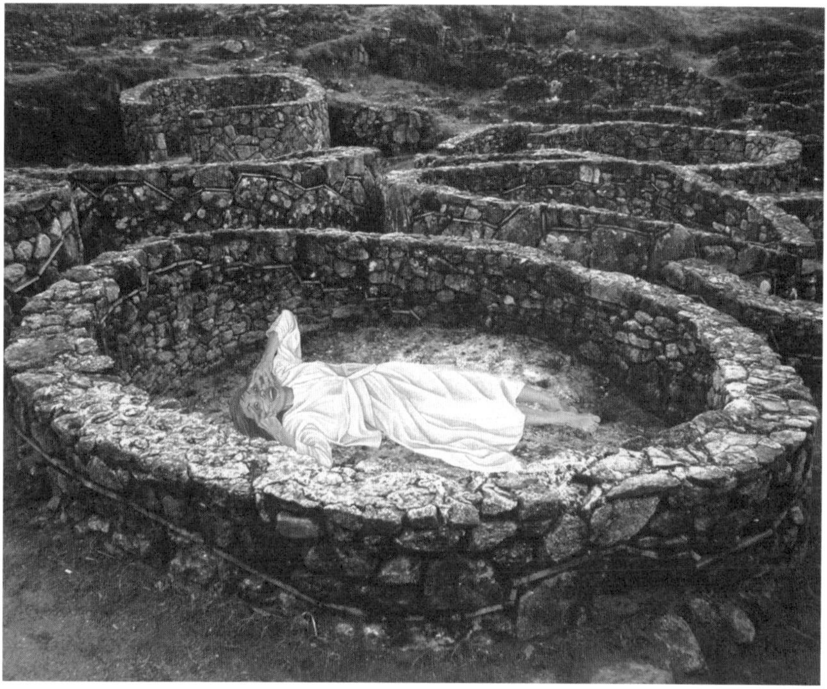

Marina Nuñez. *Locura (Madness)*, 1997.

Apart from Flaubert, Saint-Beuve or Baudelaire, there are many other authors who in one way or another confess their hysteria and link disease with creativity. Mallarmé in two of his letters – dated 4 December 1868 and 4 February 1869 – admits to having been hysterical after the several crises he suffered in his youth, which not only impeded his writing but also his speech. However, later, it appears that his bodily hysteria ended up becoming the poetic expression of his search for an idea and the means to a perfect work. Also Paul Valéry is diagnosed hysterical by his doctor. Gide, on his part, retorts in a letter dated 2 December 1894, and addressed to his friend, that hysteria is the most amusing of diseases: 'Pauvre hystérie! N'en dis pas de mal; c'est la plus amusante des maladies'.

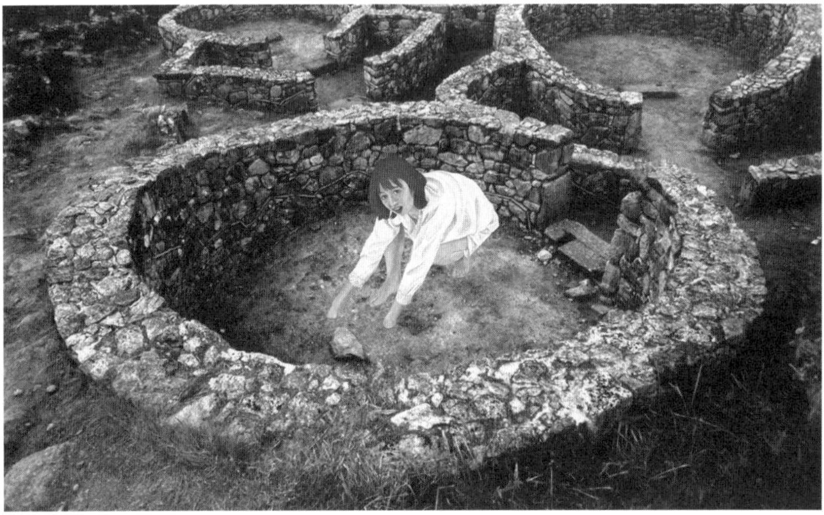

Marina Nuñez. *Locura (Madness)*, 1997.

Just as an anecdote that shows that hysteria has another face, let us remember that by that time in *Studien über hysterie*, Freud and Breuer highlighted the complex mechanisms of symbolization usually utilised by patients to elaborate their symptoms. In their line of reasoning hysteria comes to question the very conditions of creation, becoming both a brake and an engine in the artistic process. Some years later, André Breton and Louis Aragon, undoubtedly in a flamboyant manner and oversimplifying the tension between hysteria as obstacle and hysteria as energy in the creative process, define hysteria as the major poetic discovery of the late 19th century:

> L'hystérie est un état mental plus ou moins irréductible se caractérisant par la subversión des rapports que s'établissent entre le sujet et le monde moral duquel il croit relever [...]. Cet état mental est fondé sur le besoin d'une séduction réciproque, qui explique les miracles hativement acceptés de la suggestion (ou contre-suggestion) médicale. L'hystérie n'est pas un phénomène pathologique et peut, à tous égards, être considérée comme un moyen suprême d'expression. (22)

As it is, Surrealism works with psychic automatism as a tool of truth because it liberates thought bringing to the surface what lies behind consciousness. Hysteria then is the expression of psychic automatism, a mechanism that in the face of deception, frustration, aggression or suffering chooses certain symptoms to make itself understood, even though very often these are not comprehended and may lead to imbalance, mental disorder and even death.

Even today there are artists who recuperate hysteria for artistic purposes. This is the case of Marina Nuñez, who behind the plastic beauty of *Locura (Madness)* – a series of paintings based on Charcot's *Iconographie* and Géricault's pictures – communicates the rebellion, pain, strength and desire that hysteria betrays. In fact, the postures photographed by Charcot and painted by Nuñez could be interpreted as living portraits of passionate women driven by scoff, plea, vengeance, ecstasy, loneliness and angst, but, above all, driven by sexual desire because, deep down, hysteria oozes sexuality, repressed and forbidden desire. Nowadays the term hysteria has disappeared from clinical diagnoses, but its symptoms persist under the labels of conversion and dissociation disorders. However, hysteria has not disappeared as a metaphor, a mimetic and somatic mechanism of expression that despite the tragedy of illness allows artistic creation by means of the body. It survives as a tool of communication, both silent and loud, and as a space of individual freedom that releases desires and ideas because it contains creativity, liberation, repression, madness, reason, demonism, mysticism, love and sex. Hysteria is a metaphorical instrument, a language for those without language that transmutes the word into flesh.

Works Cited

Barrès, Maurice. *Un homme libre*. Paris: Perrin, 1889.

Baudelaire, Charles. *Oeuvres complètes*. Paris: Robert Laffont, 1980.

Breton, André and Louis Aragon. "Le cinquantenaire de l'hystérie." *La révolution surréaliste* 11 (1928) : 20–22.

Briquet, Paul. *Traité clinique et thérapeutique de l'hystérie*. Paris: Baillière, 1859.

Charcot, Jean Martin. *Leçons sur les maladies du système nerveux*. Paris: Delahaye, 1872–73.

— *Les démoniaques dans l'art*. Paris: Delahaye et Lecrosnier, 1887.

— *Leçons du mardi à la Salpêtrière*. Paris: Delahaye et Lecrosnier, 1887–88.

— *Leçons du mardi à la Salpêtrière*. Paris : Dehahaye et Lecrosnier, 1888–89.

— *Leçons sur les maladies du système nerveux*. Paris: Lecrosnier et Babé, 1889.

— *Clinique des maladies du système nerveux*. Paris : Babé, 1892–93.

— and Desiré M. Bourneville. *Iconographie photographique de la Salpêtrière*. Paris : Salpêtrière, 1875.

Flaubert, Gustave and George Sand. *Correspondance*. Paris: Lévy, 1904.

Freud, Sigmund and Josef Breuer. *Studien über hysterie*. Leipzig–Wien: Deuticke, 1895.

Gide, André and Paul Valéry. *Correspondance*. Paris: NRF, 1955.

Mallarmé, Stéphane. *Correspondance*. Paris: NRF, 1959–85.

Maupassant, Gilles de. "Une femme." 1882. *Chroniques*. vol. 2. Paris: Union Générales d'éditions, 1980. 111–15.

Plato. *Timaeus*. Indianapolis: Hackett, 1997.

Reynolds, Russell. "Remarks on Paralysis, and Other Disorders of Motion, and Sensation dependent on Idea." *British Medical Journal*, November 6 (1869): 483–5.

Sainte-Beuve, Augustin Charles. *Le moniteur*. Paris: Garnier-Flammarion, 1857.

Sarcey, François. *Le mot et la chose*. Paris: Levy, 1863.

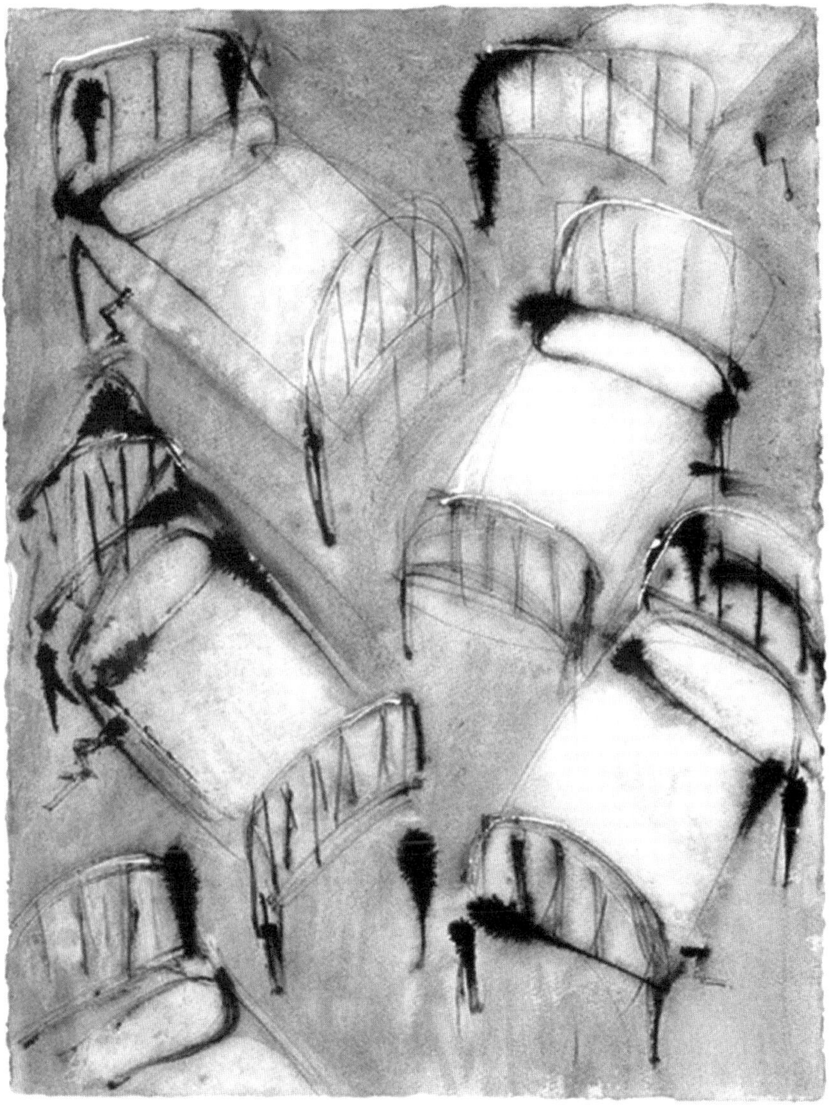

Rossana Zaera. "Habitaciones sin número" (Rooms without numbers)

Photographs as Prostheses

Nieves Pascual
University of Jaén

Pain is eternal. Pain has always been with us, and so have the attempts to contain it with representations. We all remember the images of Prometheus, condemned to suffer the peck of an eagle on his immortal liver, the stories of Loki and Job, the tragedy of Hercules, shrouded in Deyamira's tunic, and the drama of Greek Philoctetes, bitten by a snake en route to Troy. Likewise, Medea's fall to disaster, the dismembering of her brother, and the beheading of her two sons at her own hands persist in memory through Euripides, Seneca, Corneille, F. M. Klinger, Grillparzer, Hans Henry Jahnn, Corrado Alvaro, Pier Paolo Pasolini, Heiner Müllers, Ursula Haas, and Christa Wolf.[1] By domesticating pain into art they all try to make it bearable.

However true it is that nobody can suffer from you, instead of you, just as nobody can die for you, and however certain we are that pain confers identity to the individual, all representations of pain are paradoxically similar. Their likeness, Arthur W. Frank argues, is based on a "commonality of suffering (that) cuts across worlds of race and gender as well as types of disease" (170). In his book, *The Wounded Storyteller*, he examines chronic illness autobiographies, identifies the general trends and conventions peculiar to them, and proposes four kinds of narratives: The restitution narrative, the chaos narrative, the quest narrative and the testimony. Although their plots differ, all of them "have two sides. One side […] expresses the threat of disintegration […]. The other

1 See Capeola Gil's article in this volume.

side [...] seeks a new integration of body-self" (171). Be that as it may:

> People do not make up stories by themselves. The shape of the telling is moulded by all the rhetorical expectations that the storyteller has been internalizing ever since he first heard some relative describe an illness, or she saw the first television commercial for a non-prescription remedy, or he was instructed to "tell the doctor what hurts" and had to figure out what counted as the story that the doctor wanted to hear. From their families and friends, from the popular culture that surrounds them, and from the stories of other ill people, storytellers have learned formal structures of narrative, conventional metaphors and imagery, and standards of what is and is not appropriate to tell. Whenever a new story is told, these rhetorical expectations are reinforced in some ways, changed in others, and passed on to affect others' stories. (3)

Significantly, the author identifies the recurrent metaphor of being shipwrecked by the storm of disease as a defining feature in illness narratives: "The illness story begins in wreckage, having lost its map and destination" (164). For his part, G. Thomas Couser in *Recovering Bodies*, points out the existence of two other controlling metaphors drawn from the language of warfare and demonic possession. Examples abound. For Soledad Puértolas en "Locos y enfermos" pain becomes a knife, acquiring thus spatial and temporal limits (198). In *Diagnóstico Cáncer*, Mariam Suárez constructs her metastatic breast cancer as a battle against an encroaching enemy (13). Audre Lorde, an African-American woman who shares her experiences with diagnosis and later recovery in her journals, muses on the affinities which her struggle with cancer has with military war (53). In *Davalú o el dolor*, pain is metamorphosed into an Armenian devil, or else it is objectified as an army of crabs, octopuses, scorpions and reptiles so as to make it vulnerable. In this first-person narration on the suffering caused by a cervical injury, Argullol feels like a general carefully planning the battle (136). Likewise, Judith Hooper imagines her axillary lymph nodes as "alien invader[s]", and sardonically comments: "Maybe one of the cells got bored and came up with the notion of a mutiny. Screw the system! Viva la revolución!" (269).

Paradoxically these military metaphors are inherited from medical technology. As Perri Klass puts it:

> If we are at war, then who is the enemy? Rightly the enemy is the disease, and even if that is not your favourite metaphor, it is a rather common way to think of medicine: we are combating these deadly processes for the bodies of our patients. They become battlefields, lying there passively in bed while the evil armies of pathology and the resplendent forces of modern medicine fight it out. Still, there are very good doctors who take disease as a personal enemy and battle it with fury and dedication. The real problem arises because all too often the patient comes to personify the disease and somehow the patient becomes the enemy. (81)

Regardless of whether the patient or the disease are conceived of as the enemy in the medical ground, the fact is that when you contract a disease you contract the world of that disease and all its medical tropes. Still worse, in Arthur W. Frank's view, you are even "taught how to be ill by professionals" (159). And it is logical that this is so. Clearly, in all narratives of illness, a healthy voice referred to as I, now knowledgeable in symptoms, diagnoses and cures, witnesses and rationalises a former self, an other, the patient, through the residues of a medical discourse apprehended during the illness. Indeed, as Mariam Suárez alleges in her autobiography on cancer, the people who suffer from long diseases soon become doctor apprentices (92).

If the experience of pain is described as an invasion that eats the body away, a "sober banquet", in Argullol's words (35), to imagine the affected organs and the physical appearance of the empained, writers recur to alimentary products. Lymph nodes metamorphose into "pinto beans" (Hooper 109), and the patient in a bathing suit resembles "a butcher's diagram of the cuts of beef" (119). Mariam Suárez also confesses that on being told that she was a good candidate for a transplant operation she imagined herself lying face down and cut open like a cow (104). Interestingly, in *Her/She Senses Imag(in)ed Malady*, a collaborative project that Angela Ellsworth and Tina Takemoto began in 1993 when the former was diagnosed with lymphoma, Takemoto conscientiously mimics the signs of illness in her friend using marshmallows and eggs, which "begin to rhyme the shape of scars as well as the texture of the damaged skin" (121).

Clearly, there is a systematic body of prescriptions to be followed by writers. The situation of the patient before the illness is imagined as a state of pre-Fall innocence and consequently translated in biblical terms, as Dante's Paradise Lost (Suárez 114). Always it is during convalescence that the process of writing takes place. Pain has been repudiated,[2] but the narrators have not come out of the shock produced by the illness, although it is not the illness but the treatment that most traumatises.

References to the patients' obsession with reading on the illness, and the allusion to watching as a conscious antidote are customary: "Debería comer, pero no tengo hambre. Sólo tengo ganas de mirar y devorar con la mirada las imágenes. Sé que eso puede ser el mejor antídoto," [I should eat, but I am not hungry. I only feel like watching and devouring images. I know this can be the best antidote], says Argullol (84). Vision substitutes words because through vision the body decreates itself when emphasis is put on the object (Scarry 165). Consciousness of "seeing" also precipitates condensation of the logical course of time (Suárez 142).

Incompetent doctors abound and a feeling of physical, sensorial, and spiritual isolation prevails. Soledad Puértolas writes: "¡Cómo marginó la enfermedad a mi madre! […]. Veo que la enfermedad no radica sólo en la persona que la padece. Creo que

2 It cannot be otherwise because intense pain impedes speech: "Physical pain", says Scarry, "does not simply resist language but actively destroys it, bringing abut an immediate reversion to a state anterior to language" (4). Lucy Grealy writes in this respect that: "Several weeks and misdiagnoses later surgeons removed most of the right side of my jaw as part of an attempt to prevent the cancer they found there from spreading. No one properly explained the operation to me and I awoke in a cocoon of pain that prevented me from moving or speaking" (55). Later she ponders on the equation strength and silence (56). On the female insistence on suffering in silence and the usual male exhibitionism, see Bending 101.

la enfermedad ha sido decretada por esta sociedad" [How did illness alienate my mother! [...]. I see that illness does not lie in the sufferer. I believe that illness has been decreed by society] (202). The invisibility of the ill person and the infantilization or desexualization of the body in pain are further items of discussion. The assertion of physicality and the disruption of the classic mind/body duality are also recurrent. On reflecting about the prospect of reconstructive facial surgery after childhood cancer, Lucy Grealy explains: "I didn't feel I could pass up yet another chance to 'fix' my face, which I confusedly thought concurrent with 'fixing' myself, my soul, my life" (54). Precisely because the spirit is thought to be sown to the body, and the mind is forced to know itself as body, there is an emotion of shame at the suffering. However, shame often appears counterbalanced by the experience of being special and a feeling of omnipotence that results in the desire to remain wounded. Lucy Grealy hints at the bonding of victimhood with narcissism and recalls that "rather than spend all my time despairing, though certainly I did plenty of that, I developed a form of defensive egomania: I felt I was the only one walking about in the world who understood what was really important" (61). This egomania is expanded through identification with victims in Vietnam, Cambodia, Auschwitz and Birkenau. In fact, Marilyn Hacker in *Winter numbers* places her personal suffering in the context of the Holocaust and writes in her ninth sonnet: "each numbered, shaved, emaciated Jew/ I might have been. They wore the blunt tattoo,/ a scar, if they survived, oceans away./ Should I tattoo my scar? What would it say?" But as long as the rhetoric of narcissism always masks a deeper nihilism, literary references to Beckett, Sartre and Kafka abound: "As for Kafka, who had always been one of my favourite writers even before the new fashion for him, he helped me in that I felt permission to feel alienated, and to have the alienation be okay, make it bearable, noble even" (Grealy 70). Humor, serious and literal humor, is ever present as a distancing mechanism. Having being invited to give a reading at the University of Arizona,

Nancy Mairs, then confined to a three-wheeled electric scooter, recalls that:

> Having smashed three of my front teeth in a fall onto the concrete floor of my screened porch, I was in the process of getting them crowned, and the temporary crowns flew out during dinner right before the reading. What to do? I wanted, of course, to rush home and hide till the dental office opened the next morning. But I couldn´t very well break my word at the last moment. So, looking like Hansel and Gretel's witch, and lisping worse than the Wife of Bath, I got up on stage and read. Somehow, over the years, I've learned to set shame aside and do what I have to do. (276)

In view of this, there seems to be no possibility of an individual language in situations of pain. Paradoxically, to communicate about private experiences we use sensation terms that do not have as their meanings private sensations. As Hayden White wittily puts it: "the events themselves possess a 'story' kind of form and a 'plot' kind of meaning" (40). It follows then that physical pain imposes its own narrative strategies, reducing all stories to the repetition of an archaic one.

"Is it the lack of sufficient visual signs that arrests the mind in metaphoric thinking?" Takemoto wonders (110). Seemingly it is so. In effect, Lucy Grealy and Judith Hooper agree on the availability of just the aestheticized pictures of patients that "looked as if they had just come from an aerobic class" (Hooper 116), and the medical photographs: "There were gruesome pictures of people with grotesque tubes of their own skin growing out of their bodies, tubes of skin that were harvested like some kind of crop and then rearranged in ways that did not look at all normal or acceptable to my eye" (Grealy 63). Yet this counterpoint is not as contradictory as it seems because both sets of images are but "expressions of a powerful cultural mandate that individuals control their own lives" (Couser 9).

In 1991 fashion model Matuschka got cancer. In 1993 she appeared on the cover of the *New York Times* magazine baring her mastectomy: "Beauty out of Damage." Later that same year she declared that a prosthesis would allow people to forget what happened to her. Responses to the image were diverse. In Germany and France she was censored. In the United States, even though only a few pictures were published because of nudity rules, she was the recipient of honours from the World Press Foundation, the Art Director's Club, and the Rachel Carson Institute. In 1996 she was awarded the Graphis best environmental poster for the Time for Prevention Campaign created for Greenpeace: "If I didn't have the surgery," she confessed to Peter Howe, editor of *Outtakes Magazine*, "I would'nt have done this Art, and I wouldn't have been this famous, and I wouldn't have made this contribution." In her 1997 interview with Peter Schlessinger she also declared that through her photographs she aimed at overcoming the psychic wounds that resulted from the operation; she intended to pass a severe judgment on the medical profession, too prone to eliminate the problem; and claimed the need to bond illness with sex, two heterogeneous elements deliberately contrasted in her work: "I wanted to show that a woman can be beautiful, sexy, strong and powerful no matter what her body looks like."

In the 1997 picture that illustrates the interview with Schlessinger (<http://www.matuschka.net/interviews/gtgoffchest.html>), Matuschka builds a highly stylized, erotic, and androgynous body that conjures up the very idea of art. The text does not illustrate the image, rather it sublimates or rationalizes it. The operator employs the conventions of photographic art associated with femininity as spectacle and image – jewellery, make up and luminosity –: "I knew all the tricks of the trade and know my angles and poses," she confessed to Howe. The picture is taken outdoors, the referent sat on a bench "more 'alive' than indoors" (Barthes 14). Color, "an artifice, a cosmetic" (81) invades the image. The scars are hidden from sight, and the model is gazing away, not conscious of being contemplated. This indeterminate look is a typical ruse in pornography in as much as it heightens the pleasure of the voyeurs, allowing them to imagine that they are sneaking a look. In other words, the photograph is domesticated, tamed, "its

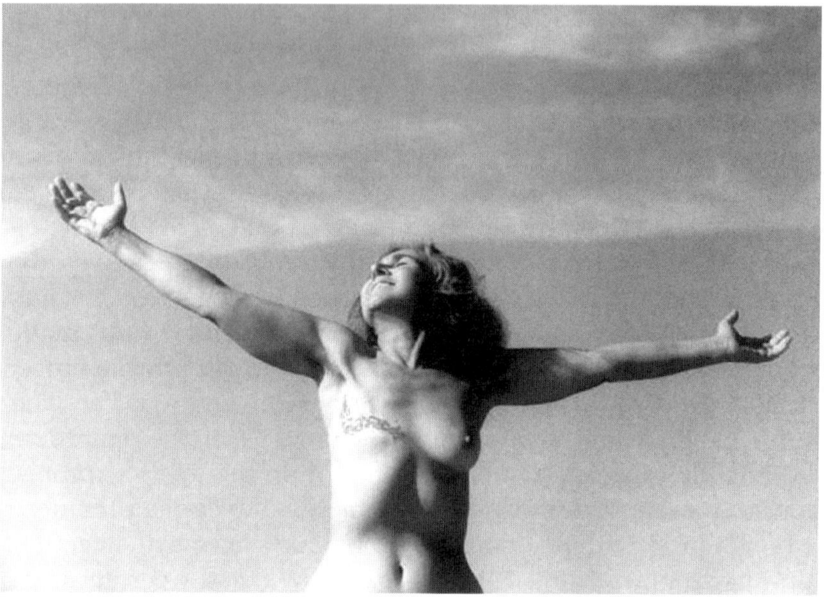

"I Am No Longer Afraid." Known as "The Warrior."
Poster. Donnelly/Colt, P.O. Box 188, Hamptom, CT 06247, USA.
Phone: 860-455-9621. Fax: 800-553-0006. info@donellycolt.com.
Design by Shiela Levrant de Bretteville (Wingbow Press, 1989).
Photograph by Halla Hammid. Copyright ©1988 by Deena Metzger.

realism remains relative, tempered by aesthetic or empirical habits" (119), "its vision [...] oneiric, not ecmnesic" (117).

However, Matuschka has no sensation of inauthenticity and imposture. She remains complicitous with the idea of photograph as mimetic mirroring and conceives of her reflection as her essential self, a double: "I state the facts [...]. I'm selling awareness and truth," she tells Schlessinger. To her it is precisely this mechanical iconicity that fosters the healing process. Seeing oneself from an objective positioning can become, in the words of Mladen Dólar, an uncanny experience that produces "the anxiety of gaining something too much, of a too-closed presence of the object" (13). In this logic, the photograph is transformed into an abstract fetish, the lost object regained, the symbolic equivalent of what is lacking, a substitute object that closes the "holed" body. In sum, it comes to be a prosthesis.[3]

Likewise, Deena Metzger takes pride in her stigmatized identity and makes the scar into art. To Elizabeth Van Schaick the tattoo she has inscribed in the place of the missing breast again acts as a fetish, a filling that replaces absence and completes her body. However true that is, by means of her tattoo Metzger also glorifies her body as unfinished, subscribing thus the socially pervasive notion that the removal of a breast makes a woman less feminine, not a whole person.

In *Multilating the Body*, Kim Hewitt explains that "[B]ody mutilation such as scarring and tattooing often functions as part of a healing ritual" (65). It signifies, she alleges, "an attempt to overcome a distressing experience" (78). Body modification, she concludes, "has become popular as modern therapy to achieve a 'manipulatable sense of well-being'" (94). So, as orthodox medicine destabilizes Metger's sense of self, she utilizes her tattoo to establish claim to her own body. On August 1, 1977, she writes on her inscription as a form of signature:

> I am no longer afraid of mirrors where I see the sign of the amazon, the one who shoots arrows. There is a fine red line across my chest where a knife entered, but now a branch winds about the scar and travels from arm to heart. Green leaves cover the branch, grapes hang there and a bird appears. What grows in me now is vital and does not cause me harm. I think the bird is singing [...]. I have relinquished some of the scars. I have designed my chest with the care given to an illuminated manuscript. I am no longer ashamed to make love. In the night, a hand caressed my chest and once again I came to life. Love is a battle I can win. I have the body of a warrior who does not kill or wound. On the book of my body, I have permanently inscribed a tree. (91)

3 To Barthes in the process of posing the individual "instantaneously make[s] another body for (myself) herself" (10).

In her examination of the internal processing of breast cancer in her life, Metzger effaces the difficulties of the disease and elevates pain to the level of an ideal, disseminating suffering as a desirable experience. Not only is pain viewed as a gift with potential for deeper knowledge of self, but it also becomes the route to strength and the activator of her creation process: "The illness I suffered was the means of profound spiritual transformation," she declared in 1997 (268).

As Van Schaick argues, the picture does not qualify as a traditional aesthetic nude because Metzger's body is not model quality, she looks active and, further, there is no subtlety about her unclothed body. Yet in its exhibitionistic relation to the camera it conveys an erotic appeal. Metzger's ceremonial posing style and her ostentatious tattoo draw the eye and contribute to its visual power.[4] Curiously, as Hewitt notes, many models have of late decided to tattoo their bodies as a fashion statement. However, as she sharply remarks, "as body modification becomes fashionable and trendy, it loses significance as a personal choice and garners importance as a cultural fad" (93). Once more, the pretence of individualism becomes proportional to the liquidation of the individual.

However different the image of Jo Spence in "Exiled" is (*Cultural Sniping*), there are striking congruities among the three pictures so far presented. All of these women are defined by a drama that explains their personality. All of them are subjects and objects of the artistic gaze, with full control over all aspects of the image's creation. They share an affective intentionality, equate the social and the subjective and erode the boundaries between the private and the public. They use the photograph as a catalyst for the new visibility of ill women and seemingly they all infringe a cultural taboo. All of them require recognition by another to confirm identity and claim the therapeutic value of photography as

4 Barbara F. Sharf explains that the details of the tattoo include grapes on a vine, *The Book of Life*, and a bird (77).

a self-discovery technique and the means of learning to accept the illness. Spence also confessed, like Matuschka, that her series *Narratives of Dis-ease* intended to level fierce criticism at the medical profession whose norms of conduct she refused to act out (*Sparerib*).

A few years after her operation in 1982, and in collaboration with doctor Tim Shears, Spence produced a series of photography works entitled *Narratives of Dis-Ease*. These five photographs trace her development as a cancer patient undergoing medical treatment. In the third photograph, "Exiled," Spence constructs her body from shame and old age. The photograph shocks and attracts revulsion, it bruises, it "pricks" (Barthes 23), because it appears to be conceived of as purely descriptive or denotative.[5] As Van Schaick argues, Spence "makes no use of traditional photographic nude aesthetics, preferring a technique approximating that of the amateur frontal snapshot." Indeed, the pictorial image seemingly offers direct access to a signified reality and transmits a non-coded, non-artificial, non-perverted, and non-travestied reality. However, only technology can simulate a non-mediated reality. Spence reconstructs the scene:

> I have a hospital gown which I stole from hospital because I needed it as a prop. I have used it in this piece of work. I then opened the gown and wrote "monster" across my chest, because that's how I experienced myself as a cancer patient: monstruous to other people: "How dare you talk about it. I can't bear to hear your pain. I might get cancer. (*Cultural Sniping* 211)

Being inscribed in the image, the text participates in this fabricated objectivity. Unnaturalness, and evilness are some of the connotations of the word "monster." Incidentally, in its semantic history, evil has long been associated with perverse sexuality. But "monster," from the Latin *mostrare*, also means to show, display or exhibit, and transmits the power of mythological beings able

5 The picture bruises the more once we know of the subsequent death of the author on 24 June 1992 from breast cancer and leukemia.

to capture vision, hypnotize the look, blind the viewers and turn them to stone.

The breast has been partially removed, and the scars, bodily memories that mediate against a complete forgetting, are visible. The body is, furthermore, parcelled out and the subject is partially decapitated and therefore, de-subjectified, destroying visual pleasure and preventing identification. What remains of the face is partly hidden behind a mask. In fact, there is no face expression to distinguish the person and authenticate her existence, and the air, to Barthes "a kind of intractable supplement of identity" (109), is certainly lacking.

Precisely because the image conforms to the myth of illness it appears to illustrate a particular medical feature, designed for the purpose of documentation or instruction. In this photograph "the female body is located not so much as spectacle but as an element in the discourse of medicine, a manuscript to be read for the symptoms which betray her story, her identity" (Doane 157). The transformation of the body into the symptom, the privacy of the background chosen, the green coat, the absence of accessories, the impossibility of recognizing the object of the gaze and the lightning bring it near a cosmetic pre-surgery photograph inviting a medical glance. However, the verbal text uproots the image from any recognizable moral framework.[6]

Like Spence, artist Hannah Wilke refuses to smooth out aesthetic deficiencies and documents the effects of the illness while it is happening and once the disease has conquered her body. This photograph is part of her posthumous exhibition "Intra-Venus" 1992–93.[7] All the images were shot by her husband Donald Goddard, but had been previously selected by Wilke for her final show. In this deathbed scene her body is veiled from view disrupting the binary notions of femininity and masculinity. She is

6 The inclusion of words also challenges the belief that an image can only communicate in a fragile and untrustworthy manner.

7 Born in 1940 she died on 28 January 1993 of complications from lymphoma.

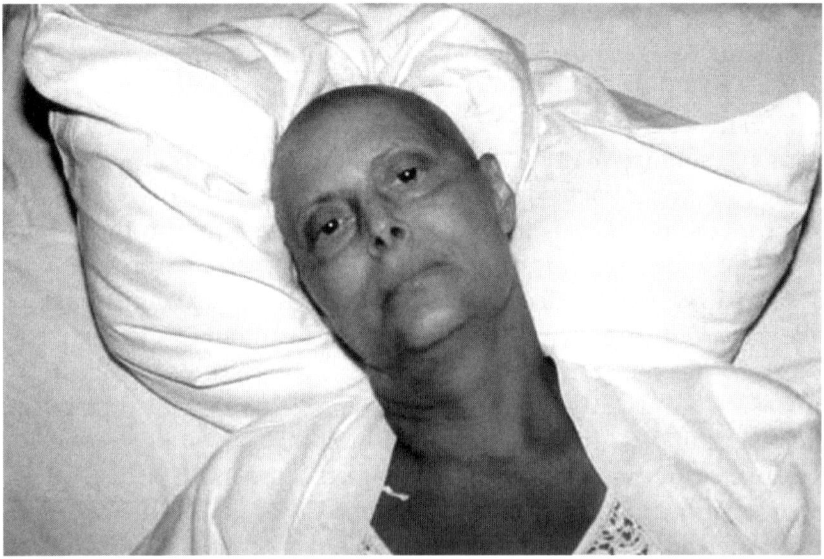

Intra-Venus Series #7, August 18, 1992, 1992-1993

depicted close-up and in full face, looking out of the picture at the viewer, but there is no threat of protest because her look is absent. Her face bears evidence of the vicissitudes of a past life and her eyes convey fears about the reality thus represented, evoking a painful awareness that life must inevitably be renounced. The image fascinates the viewers as the supreme illustration of suffering, provides discomfort and moves us to sympathy.

Although three of these images are constructed as therapeutic, they are unable to relieve the symptoms.[8] In 1986 Spence confessed: "I am not better, in spite of beginning to take responsibility for my own health." For her part, Matuschka declared in 1994: "I don´t think I am ever going to be at ease with it (my body)."

8 It seems, as Barthes alleges, that photography "excludes all catharsis" (90).

In view of their declarations it appears that photographs are not endowed with curative powers. But, do they help to relieve the suffering of the self?

Nietzsche argues that only that which never ceases to hurt stays in memory (61). Gadamer, for his part, declares that health abides by the capacity to forget (153). But, how can we forget if what feeds memory is not pain but its representation (Cyrulnik 116)? How can we forget if it is the picture that persists as opposed to the experience itself (Cameron 3)? By evoking pain, a photograph brings it to consciousness and re-enacts the experience. Within the same movement and through the re-inscription of past wounds, it becomes an act of self-injury, the protection against pain growing into a repetition of it.

But, how does the viewer create the meaning of a wound photograph during the process of perceiving it? Other women artists (Cindy Sherman, Kiki Smith, Ana Mendieta, and Gina Pane) have represented their bodies when they were devastated by chemotherapy. All of them produced either stylish pictures of health or images of pitiful illness. Although their goal was to demystify cancer, this excess of images of illness reinforces alienation and deprives the viewer of the power to react in real life. In other words, in repeatedly naming the horrors in our societies we deprive these images of their meaning and dilute the harshness of the reality they are meant to uncover. The result, as Hooper writes, is that "a lot of people have the impression that cancer is little more than a fashion" (131).

So, on the one hand, profusion fosters the erosion of the original, speeds up forgetfulness and feeds our complacency. On the other, this excess and the omniscience of the artists disempower the viewers and deprive them of agency. In fact, the artists's constant explanations about the meanings of their works in books and articles break the contract with the receivers on preventing them from negotiating meanings and symbols in their own terms.[9]

9 In this sense this essay also contributes to mitigate these images of illness.

In her interview with Peter Howe, Matuschka declared that some women objected to "the violation of their privacy. Mastectomy patients who had had a mastectomy felt that they had done such a great job concealing what it looks like, even from their husbands and now I go out and show it." In fact, women with cancer who have trouble merely coping may feel their privacy invaded and their secret deciphered.[10] If a secret made public is a social compromise, it is also true that in a culture where secrets do not exist the individual lacks reality. Significantly, Cyrulnik argues, secrets cease to exist when the individual is forced to identify with a model (170). As Grealy puts it:

> Society is no help; the images it gives us again and again want us to believe that we can be most ourselves by looking like someone else, leaving our own faces behind to turn into ghosts that will inevitably resent us and haunt us. It is no mistake that in movies and literature the dead sometimes know they are dead only after they can no longer see themselves in the mirror. (73)

Lacan's concept of the imaginary suggests that what we call the self is always a sedimentation of images we identify with. Interestingly, this process of self-identification in images have been defined by K. Myers in terms of consumption. She argues that women are defined as both the consumers of products and as consumers of themselves as commodities, i.e., as images to be consumed by the gaze of men. (137). But, as Grealy implies, in this movement of self-consumption the model also feeds upon the ego

10 This is the case in Spain. Proof of mastectomy women's disagreement with these cultural models is their support for the fashion show organised by the Asociación Española contra el Cáncer and Amoena-Coloplast Productos Médicos, S.A., held in Madrid on 19 May 2003. The 15 models had one of the breasts removed and paraded in bathing suits and underwear specially designed to support the weight of prostheses. This kind of activity is on the increase in Spain. Two other fashion shows featuring disguised mastectomy women have been presented in Badajoz (May 2003) and Málaga (June 2003) with wide acceptance.

until the latter is totally impoverished. So, in their collapse into images modern individuals disappear.

The beautification of the bodies by Matuschka and Deena Metzger certainly invite identification and consequently the expatriation of the ego toward the other subject. In addition, they may generate anxiety at the impossibility of living up to them. The pictures of Spence and Wilke, in contrast, prevent the viewer from feeling reflected in the image. They destroy visual pleasure on presenting two subjects alienated from their old, ill and undesirable bodies, and provoke fear at looking intently, but they also claim our commiseration and move us to sympathy. Significantly, Mary Ann Doane defines sympathy as "a process of contagion within the body, or between bodies, an instantaneous communication and affinity" (172). If sympathy is physiological, can symptoms be transmitted to others organically predisposed to contract them?

To Link and Phelan any state of ill-health is created and decreed by society: "Societies in part create the disease they experience and, further, they materially shape the ways in which diseases are to be experienced." They add that "the varieties of human affliction owe as much to the inventiveness of culture as they do to the vagaries of nature" (471). In this sense, Van Schaick argues that cancer is mostly a psycho-social disease. The idea, however, had already been furthered in 1917 by Georg Groddek who claimed that cancer might be produced by unconscious decisions. Just as the unconscious protects itself against chemical, mechanical and bacterial attacks, it may also produce the conditions necessary to activate pathogenic germs. In his view, this happens when certain associations of unconscious ideas or specific sensorial impressions arouse our senses of inferiority, guilt or duty. He significantly relates how scarlet fever, repressed in the most profound layers of his being, was activated on merely looking at the scarlet fever exanthema suffered by one of his patients. Although he assures the reader that contagion occurred due to his inferiority complex towards Sigmund Freud, he also concedes that the illness and its phantasm had run in his family for generations and, consequently, that he was somewhat predisposed to contract the infection (12). Had it not been for this ancestor syndrome, it would be the symptoms and not the illness itself that he simulates and produces in himself by looking.[11] Kristeva in *Powers of Horror* explains in this respect that "the theory of the unconscious [...] presupposes a repression of contents (affects and presentations) that, thereby, do not have access to consciousness but effect upon the subject modifications [...] of the body (symptoms)" (7).

Groddeck, however, is not the only one who admits to having simulated an illness. Austrian novelist Thomas Bernhard also confesses falling ill when his grandfather, whom he loved dearly, was hospitalized. The possibility of a copy-cat pleurisy is manifest upon his claiming the need to make up an illness in order to acquire conscienceness of himself and of the world around (57). But his passage from sympathy to illness is also part of his reaction against the profound fear of losing his grandfather and the need to pay homage to him. As Peggy Phelan argues, "at the heart of mimicry is the fear [...] that [...] 'the thing itself' (you, me, love, art) will disappear" (12). Likewise, the fantasy of making the self as the other is present in Eve Kosofsky Sedgwick's narration on her perception of herself after being diagnosed with breast cancer. In the section devoted to her relationship with her friend Michael Lynch, at the time sick with AIDS, she speaks about his white glasses and her "fetishistic crystallization of him through those white glasses" (253). She imitates his movements and his facial expressions. Sharon Olds, for her part, also exposes herself to the contagion "between bodies" looking at her father dying. It follows then that by looking at the last two images viewers might create in themselves some of the symptoms there imaged.

11 On simulation and dissimulation see Dana Milstein's article in this volume.

Images shape the way in which cancer is experienced in as far as "breast cancer is not just a personal process but, rather, an experience filtered through the meanings constructed by the social contexts in which women live" (Kasper and Ferguson 16). However, there seems to be a limited number of meanings from which to choose in order to respond and cope with breast cancer. The first two images presented above are produced by women with early stage cancer who erase much of the pain and suffering of the illness. The illness is optimistically portrayed as manageable, and is even imaged as a badge of honour, sending the false message that breast cancer is curable and opening the risky route to identification. If Matuschka and Metzger transform absence into a work of art, Jo Spence and Hannah Wilke, by contrast, explore their experiences with advanced breast cancer, imaged as a point of shame and equated with death. They thus induce viewers to sympathy and possibly simulation. However, despite their differences, all of them use transgression as legitimisation of order because whereas the surface plot encodes rebellion, the submerged plot reinforces social conventions and reproduces cultural images of femininity. In sum, the first two images commodify women as objects of desire, whereas the other two present breast cancer as compromising to a woman's identity, femininity and self-worth. Obviously, other models distinct in kind are required, but first it is essential to affirm individual values before we take new values from the whole.

Works Cited

Aldecoa, Josefina, comp. *Con otra mirada*. Madrid: Taurus, 2001.

Argullol, Rafael. *Davalú o el dolor*. Barcelona: RBA Libros, 2001.

Barthes, Roland. *Camera Lucida: Reflections on Photography*. Trans. Richard Howard. New York: Hill and Wang, 1981.

Bending, Lucy. *The Representation of Bodily Pain in Late Nineteenth-century English Culture*. Oxford: Clarendon, 2000.
Bernhard, Thomas. *El aliento*. Trans. Miguel Sáenz. Barcelona: Anagrama, 1991.
Cameron, Sharon. *Beautiful Work. A Meditation on Pain*. Durham and London: Durham UP, 2000.
Couser, G. Thomas. *Recovering Bodies*. Wisconsin: The U of Wisconsin P, 1997.
Cyrulnik, Boris. *La maravilla del dolor: El sentido de la resiliencia*. Trans. Gustavo González-Zafra. Barcelona: Granica, 1999.
Dólar, Mladen. "'I Shall Be with you On Your Wedding Night': Lacan and the Uncanny." *October* 58 (Fall 1991): 5–23.
Doane, Mary Ann. "The Clinical Eye: Medical Discourses in the 'Woman's Film' of the 1940s." *The Female Body in Western Culture*. Ed. Susan R. Suleiman. Cambridge: Harvard UP, 1985. 152–74.
Foster, Patricia, ed. *Minding the Body*. New York: Doubleday, 1994.
Frank, Arthur W. *The Wounded Storyteller: Body, Illness, and Ethics*. Chicago & London: The U of Chicago P, 1997.
Gadamer, Hans-Georg. *El estado oculto de la salud*. Trans. Nélida Machain. Barcelona: Gelisa, 1996.
Grealy, Lucy. 1994. "Mirrors." Foster, *Minding the Body*. 53–73.
Groddeck, Georg. *Escritos*. Trans. Ángel Cagigas. Jaén: Gráficas La Paz, 1998.
Hacker, Marilyn. *Winter numbers: Poems*. New York: Norton, 1994.
Hewitt, Kim. *Mutilating the Body: Identity in Blood and Ink*. Bowling Green, OH: Bowling Green State University Popular P, 1997.
Hooper, Judith. "Beauty Tips for the Dead." Foster, *Minding the body*. 107–37.
Kasper, Anne S. & Susan J. Ferguson. "Living with Cancer." Introduction. *Breast Cancer: Society Shapes an Epidemic*. New York : St. Martin's P, 2000. 1–22.
Klass, Perri. *A Not Entirely Bening Procedure: Four Years as a Medical Student*. New York: New American Library, 1987.
Kristeva. Julia. *Powers of Horror. An Essay on Abjection*. Trans. Leon S. Roudiez. New York: Columbia UP, 1982.
Lacan, Jacques. *Écrits: A Selection*. Trans. Alan Sheridan. N. Y.: Norton, 1977.
Link, Bruce G. & Jo C. Phelan. 1996. "Understanding Sociodemographic Differences in Health – The Role of Fundamental Social Causes." Editorial. *American Journal of Public Health* 86 (1996): 471–72.
Lorde, Audre. *The Cancer Journals*. London: Sheba, 1980.
Mairs, Nancy. "Carnal Acts." Foster, *Minding the body*. 267–82.
Marañón, Gregorio. 1957. *La medicina y nuestro tiempo*. Madrid: Espasa-Calpe.
Matuschka. Interview with Peter Howe. Fall 1994. <http://www.songster.net/projects/matuschka/interview.html>
—. Interview with Peter Schlessinger. "Got To Get This Off My Chest." 1997. <http://www.matuschka.net/interviews/gtgoffchest.html>
Metzger, Deena. *Tree: Essays and Pieces*. Berkeley: NorthAtlantic, 1977.

Metzger, Deena. *Entering the Ghost River: Meditations on the Theory and Practice of Healing*. Topanga, CA: Hand to Hand, 2002.

Myers, Kathy. *Understains: The Sense and Seduction of Advertising*. London: Pandora, 1986.

Nietzsche, Friedrich. *On the Genealogy of Morals*. Trans. W. Kauffmann and R. J. Hollingdale. New York: Vintage, 1967.

Olds, Sharon. *The Father*. New York: Knopf, 1992.

Phelan, Peggy. *Mourning Sex: Performing Public Memories*. London & New York: Routledge, 1997.

Puértolas, Soledad. 2001. "Locos y enfermos". Adecoa, *Con otra mirada*. Madrid: Taurus. 191–210.

Scarry, Elaine. *The Body in Pain: The Making and Unmaking of the World*. New York & Oxford: OUP, 1985.

Sedgwick, Eve Kosoksky. *Tendencies*. Durham: Duke UP, 1993.

Sharf, Barbara F. "Poster Art as Women's Rhetoric: Raising Awareness about Breast Cancer." *Literature and Medicine* 14.1 (Spring 1995): 72–86.

Spence, Jo." No I Can't Do that, my Consultant Wouldn't Like it." *Sparerib* 163 (1986). <http://hosted.aware.easynet.co.uk/jospence/jotext1.htm>

—. *Cultural Sniping: The Art of Transgression*. London & New York: Routledge, 1995.

Suárez, Mariam. *Diagnóstico: cáncer*. Barcelona: Galaxia Gutenberg, 2002.

Takemoto, Tina. 2001. "Open Wounds." *Thinking through the Skin*. Ed. Sara Ahmed & Jacquie Stacey. London & New York: Routledge. 104–23.

Van Schaick, Elizabeth. "Palimpsest of Breast: Representation of Breast Cancer in the Work of Deena Metzger and Jo Spence." <http://www.temple.edu/gradmag/fall98/schaick.htm>

White, Hayden. "Historical Emplotment and the Story of Truth." *Probing the Limits of Representation: Nazism and the "Final Solution."* Ed. Saul Friedlander. Boston: Lighthouse P, 1992. 37–53.

II. Restor(y)ing Pain through Life Narratives

Pain is a Preposition

Dana Milstein
Baruch College, CUNY

Jesus of Nazareth

Tweedledum, Tweedledee,
Jesus of Nazareth
complained that dying was
such a bother:

'Being nailed to that damn
cross so aggravated my
thanatophobia,
just ask Father.'

'Jesus of Nazareth' is a poem that transforms the labor pangs of Occidental culture into a tickle. Historically, Romans displayed a tortured Jesus on a cross to propagate authority. In this double dactyl, on the other hand, being crucified is reduced to mere nuisance. Suffering and dying are not glorified as a means of salvation. Pain has no value other than to assure Jesus of an impending and unavoidable death. Jesus, nevertheless, challenges his doubting listener to verify his pain with a higher authority. Only God, in spite of witnesses giving historical testimony of the torture, can confirm Christ's suffering. But when in a man's life will he speak in person with Jesus, or with God for that matter, about another man's pain and dying? Ironically, religion teaches that this dialogue takes place only after death. In a post-Nietzschean world it will not take place at all. Without God to provide concrete answers during our lifetime, how can we produce universal truths about sensing pain and feeling empathy toward those in pain?

My poem suggests that empathy itself is untenable; man's physical suffering can appear so unthinkable that it becomes implausible. Pain, whether received or witnessed, is reduced to a subjective experience that varies from one individual to another, with each person able to modify his threshold in order to achieve a desired reaction. It is the control and exhibition of our threshold that is produced for an audience. As the narrator argues in Dostoevsky's *Notes from the Underground*:

> There is pleasure even in a toothache [...] people don't suffer in silence, of course, they groan; but the groans aren't straightforward and honest, they are spiteful, and the spite is the whole point of them. The groans are an expression of the sufferer's pleasure. (24)

What Dostoevsky calls 'spite' we might call 'contrived'. A man groans, according to the narrator, to make his pain relevant. The groaner displays his customized threshold for pain by producing a moan. He derives pleasure from this artificial performance. Like the spectators of Jesus' crucifixion, witnesses to the narrator's groans 'will not believe a word of it, and they know in their hearts that he could very well groan in another, simpler fashion, without roulades and flourishes' (25). By either being acted out *by* someone, or enacted *upon* someone, pain is simulated by its dispenser to entertain a duped audience. Montaigne describes the pleasure of being duped by a production of pain:

> I sympathize very tenderly with the afflictions of others, and would readily weep to keep others company, if I could weep for any occasion whatever. There is nothing that tempts my tears but tears, not only real ones, but all sorts, even the feigned or the painted. (314)

Because pain is a production, it always requires an audience, whether as someone witnessing another person's pain, or as an individual realizing that something in his body is in pain. Unlike pleasure, pain is always given a location. A person does not say 'I feel pleasure in my ...', because pleasure, whether sexual or other, is universally described as being felt throughout the entire body.

At the same time, we do state that 'I feel pain in my…'. Feeling pain is processed as a bad sensation produced at a specific point in one's body. As witness to the pain produced 'there', we become alienated from that part because we lack the ability to create or eliminate it. We become distanced from our physical body by losing control over it – control being what most people rely on to prove their identity. Pain displaces us from our bodies and thus calls our existence into question. To reaffirm our existence, we must find a way to reclaim our estranged body. Our mind must dissimulate itself from the afflicted location over which it has no control, and produce a simulacrum of the uncontrolled pain. Jean Baudrillard differentiates between dissimulation from pain and simulating it:

> To dissimulate is to pretend not to have what one has. To simulate is to feign to have what one doesn't have. One implies a presence, the other an absence. But it is more complicated than that because simulating is not pretending: 'Whoever fakes an illness can simply stay in bed and make everyone believe he is ill. Whoever simulates an illness produces in himself some of the symptoms' (Littré). Therefore, pretending, or dissimulating always leaves the principle of reality intact, […] whereas simulation threatens the difference between the 'true' and the 'false', the 'real' and the 'imaginary'. (3)

By manipulating our threshold of pain and enacting it out as a groan, a song, a painting or other model that is then witnessed by another person, we may reestablish identity within our bodies. Pain results in an identity crisis, while the enactment of pain redefines existence.

Perhaps the text most effective for demonstrating this cycle of identity losing and reclaiming is *Oedipus Rex*. Aristotle spoke of the purpose of Tragedy, stating that:

> It is in action that happiness and unhappiness are found, and the purpose we aim at is a kind of activity, not quality […]. It is not for the purpose of presenting their characters that the agents engage in action, but rather it is for the sake of their actions that they take on the characters they have. Thus, what happens – that is, the plot – is the end for which all tragedy exists, and the end or purpose is the most important thing of all. (801)

Tragedy must focus on activity rather than a 'quality'. A 'quality', in my mind, denotes a characteristic or feeling, such as 'happiness', 'kindness', 'jealousy', or 'pain'. Tragedy cannot be limited to describing these qualities because, as Aristotle notes, 'tragedy is not an imitation of men but of actions and of life' (800). Instead of describing a character's traits, a dramatist must instead focus on how a character's sense of his defining trait is manifested. Being that 'pain' is the essential quality of any tragic hero, it is the simulation of pain that defines the action and encourages a catharsis. *Oedipus Rex* follows this cycle, which is based on Oedipus' estrangement from his pained body, his locating of that pain in a particular body part, his simulation of that pain and its implausibility to the audience, and his regaining of authority over his body and identity along with the audience's acceptance.

Sophocles's play begins with Oedipus lamenting over the unexplained sufferings of his people. When citizens implore him to find out why the land is cursed, he vouches to discover and rid the city of its unidentified corrupter, and unwittingly curses himself: 'whoever he is [...] let that man drag out his life in agony, step by painful step' (624). The audience slowly becomes aware of what Oedipus is unable to see – that he is responsible for the people's affliction because of the murder of his own father. Tiresias, who as a blind prophet cannot give plausible testimony of Oedipus's suffering, does hint at Oedipus's identity crisis by ascertaining that he is 'the murderer of the king whose murder [he] seeks' (627). Oedipus, of course, denies any allegations, and tries to invalidate Tiresias's ability by emphasizing his inability to see:

> You've lost your power, stone-blind, stone-deaf – senses, eyes blind as stone! [...]. Blind, lost in the night, endless night that cursed you! You can't hurt me or anyone else who sees the light – you can never touch me. (628)

Unlike the Chorus and other characters in the play, Tiresias suggests that what one sees is not always truth. Valid testimony can be obtained only by consulting the Gods.

Oedipus's ignorance of his true identity is lampooned by his claim to fame: he solved the Sphinx's riddle. Her riddle of the crawling, walking and hobbling entity remained unsolvable until Oedipus arrived and determined the answer as 'man'. The irony of this situation remains unchecked to most readers: Oedipus solved the enigma of mankind, and yet throughout the play remains incognizant of his own identity! The joke is further compounded by the fact that Apollo's oracle at Delphi is consulted at least three times concerning the fate of the character: Once in predicting the destruction this infant would bring upon the world if allowed to live; once just before fleeing Corinth and his 'parents', Merope and Polybus, after having been told by Apollo that he 'must make love with [his] own mother, and shed [his] father's blood with [his] own hands'; and, once when Oedipus sends Creon to discover what must be done to save Thebes. Oedipus takes the Delphic oracle seriously, and yet fails to heed the sign posted above the temple's entrance, which reads 'Know Thyself'.

What physical pain dissociated Oedipus from his body and true identity? It is not until the middle of the play that Sophocles reveals the origin of this estrangement. After having received a warning from the oracle that his son would 'strike him down', Oedipus's father Laius ordered a servant to take his three-day-old son, fasten his ankles, and fling him onto the mountains. The servant took pity on the suffering infant and left him to be found by a messenger. The messenger who discovered Oedipus as an abandoned infant is called in as a witness and the following conversation ensues:

> OEDIPUS: When you picked me up, was I in pain? What exactly?
> MESSENGER: Your ankles ... they tell the story. Look at them.
> OEDIPUS: Why remind me of that, that old affliction?
> MESSENGER: Your ankles were pinned together. I set you free.
> OEDIPUS: That dreadful mark – I've had it from the cradle.
> MESSENGER: And got your name from that misfortune too, the name's still with you. (644)

It is the pain of having his feet pinned at infancy that displaces Oedipus from his identity. He is abandoned and grows up with no recollection of why his feet are scarred, or why he carries the name 'Oedipus', which means 'swollen foot'. Throughout the play, the Chorus, his mother Jocasta, and even Oedipus himself have dissimulated themselves from the original event and refuse to accept the visible evidence of Oedipus's scarred ankles. Unknowingly, he is led to reclaim his body and control over his existence by acting his original pain out upon other characters – by murdering his father and sleeping with his mother. When Oedipus recognizes these acts, the dramatic reversal ensues, and his pathos operates as testimony for the audience. He blinds himself – an act that allows him prophetic powers like Tiresias and teaches that what we see is illusory and cannot stand as evidence. As with all productions of pain, Oedipus's act seems implausible to the Chorus. Watching his suffering, the Chorus pities him, unable to regard the terror. His distress does not answer their questions; in fact, it elicits uncertainty as to how he can bear the pain of gouging out his eyes. In their minds, it is 'better to die than be alive and blind' (653). It is not until Oedipus explains why he located his eye as the source of pain that the drama resolves itself and the lesson is learned:

> Apollo – he ordained my agonies – these, my pains on pains! But the hand that struck my eyes was mine, mine alone – no one else – I did it all myself! [...]. Don't be afraid. My troubles are mine and I am the only man alive to sustain them [...]. I with my eyes, how could I look my father in the eyes when I go down to death? Or mother so abused [...] worse yet, the sight of my children [...] nor this city either. (653–4)

Oedipus, by blinding himself, finally sees the corruption of his life, exposes his guilt in a verifiable way, dissimulates himself from his original identity, and reclaims his existence by exclaiming 'I am misery' (654). With this reestablishment, pain is no longer a preposition that is inflicted *on* and located *at* a specific point. Identity is named by one's production of misery instead of being limited to a physical location that is *in* misery.

The lesson of *Oedipus Rex* is that pain is an integral and inescapable fact of human life. The Chorus reveals the moral of the work by closing the play with '[C]ount no man happy till he dies, free of pain at last' (658). This truth can be realized only when pain is produced for an audience and inspires compassion in them. It is a cycle that one finds in many texts and artworks, to the extent that when looking through my bookshelves to consider which texts would prove my point, I laughingly questioned, 'Which one would *not* prove my point?'

In the origins of a society, pain is simulated as a 'cry', taking the form of epics that outline the major events of infant nations. Which epic poem does not begin with war, suffering, conflict and devastation? The *Aeneid* opens with 'warfare and a man at war' (*Norton* 1055);[1] *The Illiad* with 'Rage of Peleus' son Achilles, murderous and doomed' (120); *The Odyssey* with a prayer to the muse to recount the tale of 'the wanderer, harried for years on end' (225). In the Sixth Teaching of the *Bhagavad-Gita*, only control of desire, thought and action will 'destroy sorrow [...] unbinding the bonds of suffering' (1024). *Gilgamesh* begins with a wise king who 'sounds the tocsin for his amusement and arrogance, which has no bounds by day or night' (13); the *Song of Roland* with the upcoming battle between Charles le Roi and Marsilies; *Beowulf* with the death of a patriarch and the plunder of Heorot by Grendel; and *Paradise Lost* with 'man's first disobedience, and the fruit of that forbidden tree whose mortal taste brought death into the world and all our woe' (3001).

Which Ancient Tragedian does not open his works with a line devoted to one man's suffering, which then unfolds into a dissimulation from the original identity and simulation of that pain to reestablish authority? To name just a handful of the most famous: Aeschylus's *Agamemnon* begins with an inconsequential

1 Unless the works are cited in the bibliography list, all the citations are taken from the *Norton Anthology of World Literature*, vols. A–C, edited by Peter J. Simon.

servant praying: 'Dear gods, set me free from all the pain' (538); his *Eumendides* with a prophecy of murder. Euripides's *Medea* recounts a nurse's lament of the Argo reaching Colchis and bringing pain to Medea; his *Andromache* with '[I]n days gone by I was a woman to be envied, but now I am, if any woman ever was, the paragon of misery' (70). *Orestes* suggests that '[T]here is nothing so terrible to describe, or suffering, or heaven-sent affliction, that human nature may not have to bear the burden of it' (79). In Sophocles's trilogy, *Oedipus Rex* opens with the suffering people 'crying for the Healer and wailing for the dead' (617); *Antigone* with Antigone's lament to her sister of the 'griefs our father Oedipus handed down!' (658); and *Oedipus at Colonus* with 'a wandering man taught by long suffering to endure' (79).

The cycle of pain is present not only in works of war and tragedy, but also in comic texts. If one looks at *Estates Satires*, which are humorous and mocking in content, pain is often the impetus for writing these works. One notes the inherent paradox in these texts: out of pain comes great pleasure. Characters are removed from the source of their pain and placed in a pleasure dome where sex, parody and the fantastic become dominant elements. In *Estates Satires*, narrators are always people trying to escape devastation in their cities caused by plague, war, or unanticipated catastrophes. Boccaccio situates his *Decameron* in a beautiful country estate outside of Florence, which was afflicted with bubonic plague. Similarly, the storytellers of Chaucer's *Canterbury Tales* meet at an inn during a pilgrimage to St. Thomas Becket in Canterbury, in hopes that the 'blessed martyred saint, who gave them strength when they were sick and faint', will end the plague (2051). Marguerite de Navarre's *Heptameron* is fashioned when travelers are brought together at an abbey after independently encountering floods, bandits, a bear attack and murderers, which deter them from returning home. The assembly asks the eldest Lady, Oisille, to recommend a pastime that will deliver them from boredom and sorrow while they wait out the disasters. Oisille replies that 'all my life I have searched for a remedy and have found only one – the reading of Holy Scripture' (2568). Hircan, a gentleman of the group, replies that the reading of scripture relieves the soul, but not the body, of pain. His wife, Parlamente, is left to initiate a pleasure that cures their physical suffering, and she suggests that each member 'produce' a story 'either witnessed in person, or heard from someone worthy of belief' (2568). De Navarre's *Prologue* specifically outlines the production of art as a panacea for distress. *The Thousand and One Nights*, like the *Heptameron*, becomes a thread of tales woven on the loom of a man's suffering. Shahzaman and his brother, King Shahrayar, who have been betrayed by their wives and left physically ill by their deceit, decide to abandon their royal states to search for 'one whose misfortune is greater than [their] own' (1573).

One might also consider pain to be the basis of all courtly love literature. Many books have been written on the subject of pleasure (Eros, Amor and Cupido) in juxtaposition to pain and death (Thanatos). The confines of this article do not allow for a detailed discussion of this binary; nevertheless, it is worth noting the effect of pain in producing works devoted to the art of love. Borrowing from Ovid's *Ars Amoratia*, Andreas Capellanus composed his *Treatise on Courtly Love* in 1185 C.E. The text describes the pain that love inflicts on men and women, and outlines rules to be followed in simulating that pain through poetry and song. Rules 15, 16 and 23 highlight the illness that one should feel around the beloved:

> 15. Every lover turns pale in the presence of his beloved.
> 16. When a lover suddenly has sight of his beloved, his heart beats wildly.
> 23. He who is vexed by thoughts of love eats little and seldom sleeps. (14)

The butterflies in the stomach, nausea, hypersensitivity and anxiety become desirable if uncontrollable sensations inspire the ailed lover to produce song and poetry for the adored, who is witness to the courtier's suffering. Perhaps the cycle of pain is best illustrated in the closing stanzas of Arnaut Daniel's 'Art of Love':

If she does not cure me of this torment
With a kiss before New Year's
She murders me and sends herself to hell.

But this torment I endure
Could not make me turn away from loving well,
Though it holds me fast in loneliness,
For in this desert I cast my words in rhyme.
I labor in loving more than a man who works the earth
[...]. I am Arnaut, who hoards the wind,
and chases the hare on an ox,
and swims against the tide. (1808–9)

The poem begins with Daniel's estrangement from his body. According to courtly love writers, a person did not will himself to love, but rather was trapped or 'hooked' by the chains of desire.[2] Daniel is lured into love for a woman against his volition and suffers for his unrequited love with illness and a heart that 'burns and breaks apart' (1808). His identity is defined by his servitude for 'the noblest lady in the world' (1809). Like Apollo, who seizing the prize of laurel leaves off of Daphne, Daniel comes to the realization that the pain suffered by unreturned love allows for greater fulfillment in the form of poetry. By 'casting words in rhyme' (1809), Daniel reclaims authority over his suffering, sings his poem as testimony for the courtly audience and states his identity as Arnaut, a man with unconventional, Boreal powers.

With the courtly love poets and from the Middle Ages onward, pain becomes something that not only produces art, but also produces pleasure for the sufferer. Prior to this time, pain was something that was lamented, even if it did allow for the production of art that would please an audience. Oedipus, for example, laments several times that the torture he afflicted on others and was afflicted by was fated by the gods and could not be

2 Capellanus explains in a section titled 'Whence Love is Named' that '[L]ove (amor) is derived from the word "hook (amar)", which signifies "capture" or "be captured." For he who loves is caught in the chains of desire and wishes to catch another with his hook'. (9)

avoided. One senses that tragedians still tried to retain the moral idea that pain and suffering should be avoided even at the expense of art. But Saint Augustine, writing on tragedies, warned of the danger in using pain to inspire compassion in and entertain spectators:

> Whether this human agony is based on fact or is simply imaginary, if it is acted so badly that the audience is not moved to sorrow, they leave the theater in a disgruntled and critical mood; whereas, if they are made to feel pain, they stay to the end watching happily. (56)

Augustine goes on to speculate that the empathy produced in a pain-for-the-sake-of-entertainment spectacle is not genuine and even poses danger in making us desire more men to suffer so that we can produce compassion for them. Fifteen hundred years later, Dostoevsky wrote the post-script to this speculation, arguing that a bored society will concoct every kind of ingenuity to entertain itself, to the extent that golden pins get stuck into people. He goes on to divulge his worst fear: 'that for all I know people may find pleasure even in golden pins' (33).

What began as a utility to instill values and compassion developed as a necessary precondition for pleasure. By the end of the eighteenth century, revolutionaries were finding pleasure in golden pins and writers in converting political brutality into literature. The Marquis de Sade represents the archetypal figure of a man aggressed by his own society and who feeds off his physical duress to produce art. The transposition of bloodshed on the guillotine into sadistic rituals and tortures allows for what Simone de Beauvoir in 'Must We Burn Sade?' calls the 'vendetta' in Sade's writing:

> To sympathize with Sade too readily is to betray him. What he demands is that, in the struggle between irreconcilable existences, each one engage himself concretely in the name of his own existence. He approves of the vendetta, but not of the courts. We may kill, but we may not judge. (61)

Unlike his predecessors, who relied on the production of pain to generate empathy in an audience, Sade makes compassion irrelevant. The production of pain still serves a purpose in allowing man to reestablish his existence, but this restoration is not meant to be judged, appreciated, or witnessed. If Sade writes of children being raped, women sodomized and men forced into submission, it is because these fabricated descriptions simulate the pain that formed a separate existence within him. Sade subsisted through writing, and as the movie *Quills* explains, to deprive him of the quill was 'to deny him his identity and subject him to the cruelest torture imaginable'.

Similarly, Leopold von Sacher-Masoch could not have written the fictionalized *Venus in Furs* without submitting to domination by Fanny Pistor, based on a contract signed between the two on 8 December 1869. Masoch, like Sade was writing during a time when his nation's identity was being torn apart by civil revolt. Witnessing the torture and cruelty of his own people, Masoch became estranged from his society and simulated his displacement in two texts, *Venus in Furs* and its prototype, *The Estranged Wife*. Both texts devolve around a man subjected to the cruelty of a dominatrix. Unlike the reality of the political situation in Galicia, or the brutality of Fanny Pistor, the actions and experiences of the textual afflicted and inflictor are not random or involuntary. Sacher-Masoch is able in his novels to control the characters and direct the actions, thereby simulating his own pain in idealized form. The furs become a metaphor of this production: Masoch 'didn't care about contents', explains Chris Kraus in the *Foreword* to the text, 'it's the formal effect of the jacket – its *style* – that turned him on: the sexiness of power and the luxury of appearances' (xi). Fur's ability to bestow artificial elegance on its wearer became a metaphor for the pleasure of simulating pain: in Masoch's novels, the power of enacting one's pain lies in the producer's inherent deception. It is not the quality of pain, just as it is not the quality of being 'fur' that arouses pleasure. It is the action resulting from the quality – the power exercised and the result of that power over others and oneself in determining identity.

After *Venus in Furs* was completed, Sacher-Masoch attempted to put his reclaimed identity into practice by corresponding with a 19-year old aspiring novelist, Emilie Mataja. The nature of his letters to Mataja reveals an effete if established author who craves physical torture to quicken him again. As he writes in one letter, 'Physical pain by a woman predestined to me, whom I find alluring, is ecstasy. The more you mistreat me, the more I revel in agony' (36). In another letter, Masoch challenges Mataja by stating that he wonders if she will be cruel enough to allow him to visit her home. The reduplication of actual experience simulated into text simulated into a second actual experience renders the production of pain pleasurable because the 'real' pain ceases to exist. Pain, for modern writers, has lost authenticity.

Sacher-Masoch and Sade were not the first writers to speak of the pleasure in affliction. Jean-Jacques Rousseau, for example, described the delights of being spanked by his Mama in the *Confessions*:

> But when in the end I was beaten I found the experience less dreadful in fact than in anticipation; and the very strange thing was that punishment increased my affection for the inflictor. It required all the strength and my devotion and all my natural gentleness to prevent my deliberately earning another beating; I had discovered in the shame and pain of the punishment an admixture of sensuality which had left me rather eager than otherwise for a repetition by the same hand. (25)

What differentiates Sacher-Masoch and Sade from writers like Rousseau is that pain was the only medium that permitted them to write. Without experiencing displacement from their bodies as a result of the social and personal crises in their lives, neither author could have composed a single page of text.

From Sophocles to Sade, society progressed from a state in which pain was simulated in art to inspire compassion in an audience, to a state in which empathy and the audience itself was totally removed and the artist became dependent on pain as the sole vehicle of production. One might argue that the productivity of pain has taken another turn in the last one hundred years. It is no longer enough for the artist to rely on pain to simulate art. In today's world, an audience is necessary once again, but this time with the purpose of engaging spectators in the entire process of suffering along with the artist. In contemporary film, literature, and music, the audience experiences the cycle of estrangement, simulation, and restoration of its own identity. Paradoxically, and yet proving Baudrillard's point, the real no longer exists – our understanding of pain is based on an artist's simulation of his own pain, which itself might have been a simulation.

In the recent film *The Matrix*, Agent Smith explains to Morpheus, the renegade, that the first matrix developed was a utopian society. People, he claims, were so unhappy with this program that they rejected it and committed cerebral suicide:

> Did you know that the first Matrix was designed to be a perfect human world? Where none suffered, where everyone would be happy. It was a disaster. No one would accept the program. Entire crops were lost. Some believed we lacked the programming language to describe your perfect world. But I believe that, as a species, human beings define their reality through suffering and misery. The perfect world was a dream that your primitive cerebrum kept trying to wake up from.

What is important to note here is that the pain experienced in the matrix is only a simulation of pain based on a program created by the machines to duplicate their observation of human experience. Original pain no longer exists even subconsciously and those who manage to dissimulate themselves from the matrix by waking up continue to enact pain as defined by the matrix rather than by the harsh reality into which they are born. Additionally, real pain, even if it did exist, is implausible because the machines' understanding of pain was based on observation. As Mouse, the nihilist character of the film, points out:

> Now how did the machines know what Tasty Wheat tasted like, huh? Maybe they got it wrong. Maybe what I think Tasty Wheat tasted like actually tasted like, uh […] Oatmeal or Tuna fish. That makes you wonder about a

> lot of things. You take chicken for example. Maybe they couldn't tell what to make chicken taste like which is why chicken tastes like everything!

Just as the machines might have muddled the taste of Tasty Wheat through lack of direct experience eating it, so also the fact that they based their understanding of human suffering on an enactment of pain allows us to speculate that what they witnessed was itself modified.

Film and music of the twentieth century best prove that metasimulation is preferable to simulating a real experience of pain. Whereas the latter tends to produce false compassion and empathy in an audience, the former actually induces anxiety and paranoia in spectators and forces them to experience pain as well. One has only to consider Salvador Dali and Louis Buñuel's *Un Chien Andalou* to grasp this concept. The film opens with a note that this is a *mise en scène* of a scenario previously created by Dali and Buñuel. Already the directors are signposting that the scene is a simulation of a preconceived scenario, which itself was probably based on an actual experience. It proceeds with the passing of a sharpened razor through a woman's eye just as a sliver of cloud moves across the face of the moon. The razor simulates the moving cloud, which in turn is a simulation of the director's destroying of the visible, illusory world in favor of the subconscious and dreams, which are authentic. Jean Vigo, in the *Foreword* to the 1930 film transcription, writes that:

> Our cowardice, which leads us to accept so many of the horrors that we as a species commit, is dearly put to the test when we flinch from the screen image of a woman's eye sliced in half by a razor. Is it more dreadful than the spectacle of a cloud veiling a full moon? (xxv)

The film evokes terror in the audience by creating double and multiple reproductions of events based on this initial scene. The initial scene itself is displaced because the film is unfaithful to chronological order and randomly jumps from past to present throughout. In the next sequence, one shot of a man riding his

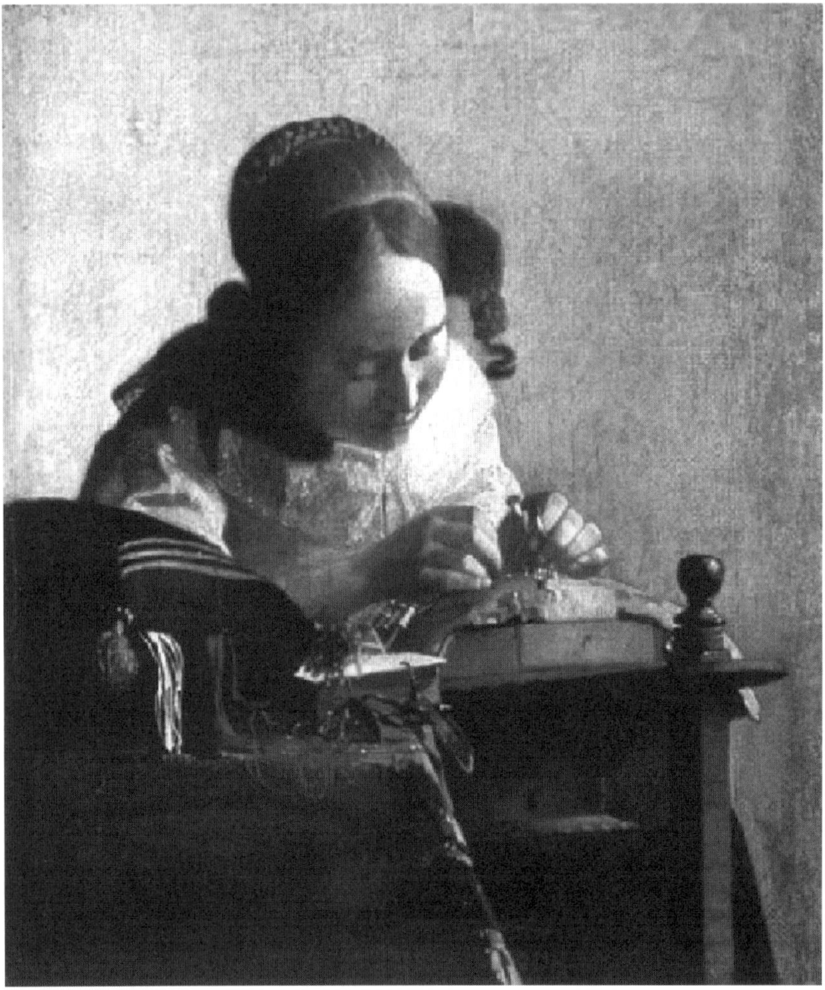

Johanes Vermeer. 'The Lace Maker' 1669–70

bike and wearing a striped box is superimposed on another shot of the street on which he is seen cycling from behind. An additional miniature slices through these superimposed images, which seems to be a footage taken of the superimposed shots. The effect is unsettling, in that the viewer becomes totally unable to discern between the actual cycling event and the filmed footage of the event – all of which, of course, we must remember are fictionalized events in a directed film. Following this scene, a woman sitting in her apartment and absorbed in reading suddenly stands and throws her book onto a nearby couch, where it remains open to a reproduction of Vermeer's *The Lace Maker*. The painting was actually a replication of an image that Vermeer made in 1669 using a camera obscura on a live worker. Interestingly, using this tool often resulted in the blurring or mis-shaping of objects in the foreground. Vermeer's painting, then, is based on the inaccurate testimony of his reproduction. At any rate, the woman runs downstairs after witnessing the cyclist topple over, and the scene is submerged in a torrential rain that blurs the film. The camera focuses on the box, whose diagonal stripes slowly become superimposed on the diagonal lines of falling rain. The rain, the box, the tissue paper and the tie contained in the box form a pattern of diagonal stripes until the woman removes the tie and lays various items of clothing on her bed as they appeared on the cyclist, who then shows up no longer wearing the items laid on her bed. No additional description is needed to guess where the film is going – all the events become simulations of scenes that appear earlier in the film, which in turn overlap *pre*ceding scenes, since the movie is not filmed in linear chronology. Events slice through each other just as the razor sliced through the woman's eye. The duplicity does not produce compassion, but rather initiates paranoia and anxiety in the viewer who is desperately trying to determine which was the authentic scene that gives this film its identity.

I never once winced, or felt anxiety or paranoia during the many times I watched *Un Chien Andalou*, and admittedly I always wondered why my students and peers were so traumatized by it. Last month, however, I was invited to a viewing of the Indie film *Irreversible*, which allowed me to experience first hand an artist's use of simulated torture to initiate a cycle of pain within the audience. The movie opens with the camera moving in circular, frantic motions on the dark wall of a building as the sound of a revved engine or buzzing fly fades in and out. Before any action or conversation ensued, the viewer begins to experience vertigo and nausea, already displacing authority over one's body. The camera hones in on two old men, seemingly ex-cons, one who is recollecting his adoration and incestuous abuse of his daughter. He verbalizes the moral of the film, '[T]ime destroys all things'. A siren has been sounding throughout their discussion and comes to the fore as the spinning camera shifts out of focus and takes the viewer to street level, where a woman is being loaded onto an ambulance. The premise of the film is that a beautiful, pregnant woman leaves her boyfriend at a party, and falls victim to rape in an underground passage, where she is brutally sodomized and beaten unconscious by a man who mistakes her for a 'dirty whore'. The events unfold counterclockwise, and two extremely graphic and disturbing scenes occur.[3] In the first, the boyfriend and her former lover enter an underground gay bar, where men are caught on tape performing S&M and bondage, masturbating, drinking and cavorting. The viewer is given only glimpses of the scene because of the rotating camera, but the vertigo effect situates us in the club as one of the many drunken voyeurs. Finding the man they believe to be the rapist, the former lover beats the man to death with a fire extinguisher. The battering is detailed to the extent that we witness the skin being burnt and peeled off the face to reveal bone, which is then smashed inward piece by piece as the man gasps for air. The scene was so vivid that many members of the audience stood up and left at this point. Later in the film, which is earlier in the story, the ten-

3 This reversal of chronological events is now common in films, including *Un Chien Andalou*, *Memento*, *Pulp Fiction* and *Rules of Attraction*.

minute rape is filmed head on. The movie arrived at its terminus, which depicts the beginning – the happy mother-to-be reading in a park with children dancing in a circle around her, and that circle spinning up like a cyclone into the clouds as programmatic music belts out. I felt completely displaced, having experienced, as the movie critic Neil Young described, 'a sensory assault that begins with the first frame of the opening titles, and continues to the retina-blasting, eardrum-pounding coda 95 minutes later'. As a female forced to watch this seemingly endless struggle, I transferred the simulated rape into my own feeling of being violated by the director. I had the feeling of belonging nowhere, and had no desire to do anything other than walk aimlessly around the city. In my mind the rape scene was a real event and for three weeks it haunted me in moments of solitude – on the train, during work and lying in bed – causing me to feel nausea or break down in tears or shivers.

Last week, and perhaps in the writing of this paper, I was able to simulate the pain that had infected me by composing a new song for my album. Music has been my escape from pain since childhood, and in the past two years I started writing and recording my own material. Most of my songs trace the frustration of unreturned love, or the guilt of hurting others at the expense of personal advancement. I find myself most inspired when my desires are least fulfilled; in other words, when lack motivates me to produce something to fill in the empty gaps. Watching *Irreversible* resulted in three weeks of estrangement from my body, but I was able to reclaim authority over pain by defining my experience of it in 'Lover's Lullaby 9–11'[4]:

> You needed me to sing you a lullaby
> To help you get to sleep tonight
> Took ashes from the memories in your mind
> To light this vigil for you

4 Clips of this and other songs, as well as biographical information, photos and general discography can be accessed at www.daynblakeley.com.

Have to find a way to guide you back
To the place where time can't last
And questions don't need an answer
That satisfies our peace of mind on this path

(chorus) And maybe misery's the elixir of life
Pushing us ever forward
I can't imagine what death would be like
Guess to have all that we wanted

I hate the empty smiles on the street
I hate the cautious winds in the air
I miss the sticky feel of our touch
When trains weren't packed with vacant stares

We always need a scapegoat to blame
Someone to bear the burden of all our shame
Could have been me or your best friend
Guess we have to turn on us all in the end

So what does it matter if we're wise
We're still dust beneath the beggar's feet
Who drinks for thirst, eats for hunger
And hears the unexpressed fears in us all
Close your eyes
Kiss me and don't let go
You don't need ephemeral recognition
Or that house on the hill or that car
Give it all up
Breathe
Enjoy the day
And just live

As the opening of the song suggests, an event had displaced me, and I needed to be guided back to my identity. The chorus defines life in terms of pain – without it, humans have no motivation to progress. Happiness, on the other hand, is complete stasis and the death of desire. The middle two verses describe how most humans respond to estrangement from their bodies: We become suspicious, vacant and alienated not only from ourselves, but also from other objects that we see as the inflictors of our suffering. We enact that pain by creating scapegoats who in turn we victimize to transfer our suffering. The closing verse points out that enacting pain through materialism, artifice, victimization, or rationalization of our emotions is pointless. Instead, we must abandon our artificial simulation, return to reality, and live our lives to the fullest in spite of random experiences of pleasure or pain. Completing the song, I added the subtitle '9–11', because much of my own pain and estrangement of late has been the result of observing my husband's post 9–11 trauma, when he returned home covered in ash as one of the thousands trapped in the World Trade Center after the second plane crashed, the buildings crumbled and pedestrians perished as a result of heart and asthma attacks, or falling debris. Since the song is titled 'Lover's Lullaby', the music behind my lyrics needed to be sweet and sad, just as the lullabies that our mothers sang to us as children to comfort us into slumber. Many lullabies and fairytales prove that narrating pain can lead to peace and security for the listener.

Pain, unlike pleasure, is a quality that posits a cycle of productivity. Pleasure is an end in itself, while pain is only the beginning of identity formation. It is interesting to imagine a utopian world where pain is eliminated and pleasure prevails. Easily enough I can imagine a tickle caused by a small spider crawling along my neck, or an orgasm produced by focusing on the pulse in my erogenous zones. I cannot, on the other hand, imagine that the same spider is boring a hole into my neck, or that my arm is on fire. I cannot, and most people cannot, produce something along the lines of stigmata. The paradox of human life is that we rely primarily on pain to produce art and yet it is the one thing we are unable to self-produce. If we are to perpetuate art along with human progress, we must do as Rilke advises. We must 'think that something is happening with [us], that life has not forgotten [us], that it holds [us] in its hand, that it will not let [us] fall' (70). We must not shut out any agitation, pain or melancholy because, as Rilke points out, how do we know what these states are working *upon* us? Pleasure is a noun that we create internally. Pain is a preposition that is inflicted *upon* us and dissimulates us *from* ourselves. Pain is the cycle that rocks our cradles, forces us to fall and leads us to stand tall in the face of Beauty.

Works Cited

Aristotle. *Poetics*. Trans. S.H. Butcher. New York: Hill and Wang, 1961.
Augustine. *Confessions*. New York: Penguin, 1961.
Baudrillard, Jean. *Simulacra and Simulation*. Trans. Sheila Faria Glaser. Ann Arbor: U of Michigan P, 1994.
Beauvoir, Simone de. "Must We Burn Sade?" Introduction. Sade, *The 120 Days of Sodom and Other Writings* 3–64.
Buñuel, Luis. *Un Chien Andalou*. Trans. Phillip Drummond. London: Faber and Faber, 1994.
Capellanus, Andreas. *Art of Courtly Love*. Trans. John Parry. London: Continuum International Publishing Group, 1983.
Dostoevsky, Fyodor. *Notes from the Underground*. Trans. Jessie Coulson. New York: Penguin, 1972.
Euripides. *Andromache and other Plays*. Trans. David Grene. Chicago: U of Chicago P, 1958.
— *Orestes and other Plays*. New York: Penguin, 1976.
The Matrix. Sounds and citations provided online. <http://www.moviesounds.com/matrix.html>
Kraus, Chris. Foreword. Sacher-Masoch, *Venus in Furs* v–xi.
Montaigne. *The Complete Essays*. Trans. Donald Frame. Stanford: Stanford UP, 1976.
Rilke, Rainer Maria. *Letters to a Young Poet*. Trans. M.D. Herter Norton. New York: Norton, 1993.
Rousseau, Jean-Jacques. *Confessions*. Trans. J. M. Cohen. New York: Penguin, 1953.
Sacher-Masoch, Leopold von. *Venus in Furs and Selected Letters*. Trans. Uwe Moeller. New York: Blast Books, 1989.
Sade, Marquis de. *The 120 Days of Sodom and Other Writings*. Trans. Austryn Wainhouse and Richard Seaver. New York: Grove, 1966.
Simon, Peter J., ed. *The Norton Anthology of World Literature: Beginnings to 1650*. Second Edition. 3 vols. New York: Norton, 1984.
Vigo, Jean. Foreword. Buñuel, *Un Chien Andalou* xxv–xxvi.
Young, Neil. *Irreversible*. <http://www.allmovieportal.com/m/2002_Irreversible26.html>

Sleep's Guile: Insomnia and the Work of Art

Eluned Summers-Bremner
University of Auckland

> Pain: the coupling of the external and internal, of reality and phantasy, of the past and present. This tight embrace is difficult to undo.
>
> J.-B. Pontalis, "On Psychic Pain" (205).

Pain is a phenomenon at the threshold of representation, where the body, once subdued by the demands of common language, reverses itself, where the words and images through which bodily reality is ordinarily filtered, simplified and grasped as experience are sundered by affective overflow. Radically unmastered, the subject in pain is caught between at least two inter-related orders, that of the human as organism and that of the human as communicant or social being. Pain registers on the one hand as physical excess, a saturation of somatic signals fighting for recognition. Language, consequently, becomes strained and depleted, as the interplay of internal and external forces by means of which affect is routinely, albeit arduously, transformed into social code and rerouted to the site of an internal casualty, a crisis in the relation the subject has with him- or herself. Pain takes us out of the communication loop and into the linguistic and symbolic borderlands. If it is characterised by one particular desire or impulse, it would be the wish to escape pain, to return from exile to the everyday where body is a passage to the world again, an unconsidered dream of colloquy and completion.

Writing about pain, even in response to or accompanied by its peculiar mode of chaotic registration, cannot, thus, ever quite convey its complex character. While it is undoubtedly the case that the attempt to come to terms with pain's imperspicuity offers the world at large, and the individual, aesthetic and symbolic benefits – the work of art, like pain itself, accruing value at least partly through its mystificatory status, its tangential relation to mechanistic codes of production – pain and the production of the work of art are not quite bedfellows. Aesthetic labour can certainly be painful, yet by and large is registered as a gain, and thus as resulting from a degree of mastery or symbolic recapturing of suffering, whereas pain itself, as Elaine Scarry has famously argued, reduces the representational to its aversive ground: sheer alienation (52). If the everyday or optimal operation of embodiment is, as I described it a moment ago, something of an easy dream, the subject's ability to take motility, expansion, conversation and quietness for granted (rather as one takes the screen that supports a dream's scenography and action for granted while dreaming), then pain, where the body is severed from meaning, and from meaning's conveyances, is unsought wakefulness.

What then of that state of mind and body which, when enforced by another, can be torture but which, seemingly unenforced by the sufferer upon him or herself, and thus not quite qualifying as pain, nonetheless courts pain as prospect, sometimes heralding it or speeding its arrival, and, at least, annihilating recuperative oblivion: insomnia? What is the relation of sleeplessness, a kind of trial run at pain, a threshold state with its own peculiar terrors and nuances, discomforts and distortions, to the processes of production of the work of art? If pain is self-sundering in a way that requires all one's energy and more, taking the sufferer to and beyond the limits of self-containment, and if aesthetic production is, among other things, a retroactive accommodation of pain's event, might insomnia not be a best (or worst) of both worlds scenario, a kind of middle way between the enforced self-sufficiency of pain, which occludes the sufferer, and the self-consciousness of art, which occludes the arbitrary and suffers, if anything, a surfeit of meaning?

Insomnia is a moment where the self, if not exactly in pain, is nonetheless troubled by the extent of pain's reach and jurisdiction. It is precisely the inability to trust the night, and rest, and sleep, that keeps the insomniac wakeful. An unwilling interrogation of night's benignness, insomnia stalks the sleepless like a rogue demon queen, enlisting supporters in a mission of watchfulness, inducing doubt in the valency of any number of commonplace distinctions that order and make sense of the world: night/day, dream/reality, hope/fear, sanity/insanity, and, perhaps most freighted of all for the artist, creativity/sterility. If I were to be offered the choice between sleeping well forever or continuing to be able to fall, apparently at will yet at the same time revivingly into writing, I would choose sleeper's over writer's block ('better the devil you know…') every time, no question.

In this essay I want to consider insomnia as a figure for the conundrum of the restorative occlusion that gives value to writing and sleeping. Artistic creativity is understood as active labour in part through its withdrawal from the world in response to a muse or other (seen or unseen) collaborator. There is in its work an unavoidable element of secrecy or hiddenness, if only the hiddenness of the work's value, during making, to the maker him or herself. Pain, conversely, is understood as passivity to the extent that it enlivens the sufferer beyond the point of manageability or requires language to revert to its most fundamental task: to mediate between self and world at the point where the body requires not only physical aid, but translation. 'By speaking, pain becomes suffering', as Harold Schweizer notes, 'acquiring a narrative, cultural dimension' (Schweizer 230). In its needful encounter with speech and language, pain yields up its privacy and language gains its visceral or heartfelt qualities, perhaps its ultimate meanings.

If language both translates and depends upon the body's tendency to encounter pain as excessive and to seek mediation, then literature, the field where language claims the right to expand or alter the consciousness of human beings, in turn depends upon a contract with the suffering or seeking reader, one that is largely carried out in private. The seeming arbitrariness of suffering – the realization that follows pain's passage into language (the 'what now?' aspect) – can become, in the act of reading and writing, something greater – an attribute of citizenship or humanity – on the condition that it becomes something less: the heightened or acknowledged pain of a singular, perhaps ultimately incommunicable, existence. Where insomnia meets literary creation is at the point of admission of the fundamental arbitrariness of being human, where to sleep, or speak, is to fall into common rest or common language, only knowable in such democratic, and thus incontestable, terms.[1] To write for an invisible community or to court the invisible succour of nightly rest is to encounter what Jacques Lacan would call the *extimité*, or intimate alterity, of our uniqueness (Miller 1988). To speak or write at all is to accommodate a rupture of the symbolic code enabling speech, just as to chase sleep is to consent to fall out of the jurisdiction of the day whose terms provide the only meaning we can know, and to momentarily inhabit the self-vacating space of our own desire whether for soporific or writerly communion.

Insomnia is, if nothing else, the sustaining of a tensile moment between two states, and is not unrelated to the contradictions of literary inspiration, whose Latin etymology carries the sense of breath and voice, and the powerful displacements that the voice can bring to the act of communication (Clark 3; also Connor 2000). 'Inspiration is held to blur conceptions of agency', as Timothy Clark observes: 'the writer is possessed or dispossess-

1 As Joan Copjec details, after Claude Lefort, the subject of both Lacanian psychoanalysis, in its theory of language, and democracy is the 'non-substantial subject of the unconscious' in the sense that democracy makes possible the expression of a range of human desires on the condition that it not privilege any particular one: 'the empty place of democracy [...] is a place of nonsense, the place where a signifier is lacking. The empty place "also" gathers all the people, but not the people in general; rather it gathers them one by one, in their "distributive exhaustion"' (57).

ed', while 'agency is uncertain and mobile – we speak of an inspired text, without reference necessarily to an author' (13). To the extent that inspiration depends upon the risk of dispossession, its companion would seem to be not insomnia but sleep, where the self is routinely inhabited by its other, the unconscious in the mode of dreaming. And if insomnia is the border land where these two selves debate the respective benefits of sleeping and waking, their literary correlative is the page or screen, whose constructive role in the work of inspiration is similarly incircumscribable by writer and reader. Its material opacity, like the conduct of the body in the act of sleep, performs the function of conveyance between worlds, and can thus give rise to anxiety regarding the writer's or the sleeper's obsolescence.

Insomnia, like writer's block, is nothing if not anxious. 'Where do we go when we sleep?' asks the American poet Edward Hirsch, 'and how do we wake up again and remain just one person when so many others shuffle through our restless minds at night?' (60). 'Hence', Hirsch writes, 'the title poem of my first book in which I turned sleepwalking into a mysterious, metaphysical act of trust', akin to the raid on the inarticulate that is poetry:

> I love the way that sleepwalkers are willing
> to step out of their bodies into the night,
> to raise their arms and welcome the darkness,
>
> palming the blank spaces, touching everything.
> Always they return home safely, like blind men
> who know it is morning by feeling shadows. (60)

There is a considerable history of the relation between insomnia and literary creation, nonetheless (Fontana 1990; Messer 1996; Deagon 1998; Spaar 2000). And as Jane Messer reminds us, while the insomniac is 'separated from other good citizens by the affliction [...] we must be careful not to always regard it as suffering' (Messer xv; also Deagon 466–7). Indeed, writers can become positively addicted to the opportunities insomnia offers, not only a relatively uninterrupted expanse of time in which to work but a quality that is becoming increasingly rare in the modern world of continual destruction and rebuilding: relative quietness. The quietness of night is, of course, variable – a number of turn of the century writers, for instance, treat insomnia as a logical result of the perpetual stimulation offered by the modern city (Thomson 1910; Kafka 1994; Rilke in Messer 1996). Yet, in its long-time association with dreaming as divine inspiration and symbolic elaboration of the day's excess, night time quietness is an absence charged with fullness, an overdetermined time and space in which the recuperation of energy and a readying for daytime's onward passage through civility concur.

Night time quietness is a state of mind and body encompassing more than the absence or relative mutedness of sound or of stimulation by sight. At night the senses are sharpened even as the body seeks repose. The ancient evening service of prayer known as Compline performs the double act of soliciting divine protection from the evils that walk abroad in darkness while at the same time joining with others in an act of nightly vigil. In echoing the distinction between life and death – the final sleep, or perhaps the final torment – the liturgical passage from day to night is a reflection on the centrality of paradox to Christian tradition, in which the tomb begets new life and in which dying to individual desire enables, ideally, a greater comprehension of those desires shared by all. The demons that stalk the night hours may imperil the wakeful but less so, it is hoped, to the extent that the wakeful or the sleeping admit the vexed passivity of night, not only its theological history as the battleground of good and evil but more centrally, perhaps, its supreme unknowingness, its harbouring of human vulnerability or potential for a trustful praxis. It is this orientation towards dispossession or perpetual journeying that leads Hirsch to characterise sleepwalking as the act in which 'our hearts are leaving our bodies' (60), as they are also said to do in the act of love, whether as *amour* or charity, a recognition of sleep's – and love's – fundamental hopefulness or lack of guile.

And it is in this indeterminate yet expectant zone that the writer and the insomniac join forces, for both are engaged in an encounter with the invisible whose imaginary presence is summoned by the shadows and relative soundlessness of night. For the writer, it is the reader who must be posited – even if it is only the reader of her own work that the writer is yet to be – in order to sustain the work of writing. For the insomniac, there is an equally necessary task of conscious or unconscious supposition, requiring similarly taxing levels of credulity. Simulating disinterest – indeed, simulating the most infantile state of unknowing dependence – the insomniac seeks the company of a friend that she will never see or know, and whose succour can never be measured and so never brought completely within the purview of acknowledgement, of conscious debt or gain.

Sleep is a friend who may just as well, for all we know, be an enemy, as it was for *Macbeth*'s Duncan. Yet as the end of life approaches, this muse is wished for as the sleep of death (a happy way to go), our greatest foe becomes an intimate through sleep's kind mediation. Perhaps it is the kinship between sleep and mortality and the paradoxical illumination of that most mysterious of states suggested by its likeness and unlikeness to sleep that the insomniac writer senses, and, sensing, cannot but desire to know further. 'The poetic insomniac', as Hirsch describes him or her: 'is one who takes the romantic connection between sleep and death a little too seriously' (61). Stranded on the faultline between trust and experience, control and abandon, the insomniac, at least, like the writer, renews a contract with blankness or absence of communication as communion and with communicative passage (the night, the page, the screen, the sleepwalk, the dream, the journey) as oblivion.

The romance of the road, or, fear of falling

> Merely to breathe was enjoyment; and I derived positive pleasure even from many of the legitimate sources of pain.
>
> Edgar Allan Poe, 'The Man of the Crowd' (in Messer 203).

The writer, as Maurice Blanchot conveys so well, is routinely inhabited by the vexing sort of pain that is both tempered *and* augmented by writing, which is another way of saying that writing is highly addictive. Blanchot gives this painful state of mind and body the name of a condition that can take an object but, if necessary, can suffer just as long and hard without one: he calls it the writer's dread (1999). As a result of the fact that

> there are, in the world, men who have pushed the art of signs to the point of language, and concern for language to the point of writing [...] the case of the writer has something exorbitant and inadmissible about it. It seems comical and miserable that in order to manifest itself, dread, which opens and closes the sky, needs the activity of a man sitting at his table and forming letters on a piece of paper. This may well be shocking, but in the same way that the necessary condition for the solitude of a madman is the presence of a lucid witness. The existence of the writer is proof that within one individual there exist side by side both a man full of dread and one who is cool and calculating, both a madman and a reasonable being, a mute who has lost all words firmly wedded to an orator, master of discourse. (346)

In the person of the writer, Blanchot claims, dread is represented in a particular way, simultaneously challenging the powers of reason – dread, after all, tends to sit, unmoved by argument, in the pit of the stomach like a stone, a deadweight – and summoning them at the same time. The writer 'remains attached to discourse; he departs from reason only in order to be faithful to it; he has authority over language, and he can never completely send it away' (346). This situation should not, he goes on to argue, 'be confused with the sterility that sometimes overwhelms an artist', for even when 'his whole mind is language', as a bird to the sky or a fish a stream, 'the exercise of [the writer's] power forces him to sacrifice that power' continually (347). 'Work', Blanchot suggests, or writing work at least, is only 'temporarily possible in the impossibility that weighs it down' (350).

In part, Blanchot is detailing here the impossibility of comprehension or clarity in the relation the writer has with his or her work, that maddening property through which one's own writing appears, in bleaker moments, as all privacy, a shambles of inadequately translated meanings, of stabs in the dark, only to appear, once successful, unrecognisable to the writer as her own. The hit the writer feels on encountering evidence of her own writing's quality is double edged: as soon as the writerly aim has been achieved, the result appears to the writer as the work of someone who has plainly never suffered the merest smidgen of a lack of facility with words. The very ease with which the words of the finished text convey a fit between the writer and her evident purpose occludes the reality of the writer's barren day or page as the day itself does the meaning of the insomniac's sleepless night. To the extent that the writer continues on the path of pushing words about to make a world whose life is fostered by the book, the work that has achieved this end disappears into the world of other words and other books, of bookish adulthood, whence it returns to the writer as from a foreign shore or city, an alien instance of sophistication. The writer, like the parent or the teacher, has no recourse: from now on, her work will only ever be the work of someone else.

Blanchot's own thoughts on sleep – like writing, an act of consummate solitude inseparable from a required communion (night time is the time when all should sleep) – go further than this and suggest that the literary work's worklessness is related to the absence from ourselves that we practice when we are sleeping. Blanchot describes sleep as an act of faith in its own beneficence and sleeplessness, by extension, as suspicious both in action and appearance: 'People who sleep badly always appear more or less guilty. What do they do? They make night present' (Blanchot 1982, 265). If sleep is 'inattention to the world', it is a benign negation whose practice results in affirmation:

> Sleep belongs to the world; it is a task. We sleep in accord with the general law which makes our daytime activity depend upon our nightly repose [...]. There is between sleep and us something like a pact, a treaty with no secret clauses, and according to this convention it is agreed that, far from being a dangerous, bewitching force, sleep will become domesticated and serve as the instrument of our power to act. We surrender to sleep, but in the way that the master entrusts himself to the slave who serves him. Sleeping is the clear action which promises us to the day [...]. Only deep sleep lets us escape what there is in the deep of sleep. Where is night? There is no longer any night. (264)

In this understanding, both sleep and writing are characterised by a working absence, the absence of care on which depends a facility with words or sleeping. Insomnia, by contrast, is all care, and thus related to the condition known as writer's block where the writer is not so much suffering from a lack of words as from a lack of discernment or inspiration. In this overheated state words crowd in, each as useless and nugatory as each other. The page or screen suffers the equivalent of a word headache, or a word famine ('Which words to use? No words are better than the wrong ones...'). In this respect a writing block is perhaps best described as a forced encounter with the mass culture, the fearsome democracy, of words, words as a barricade to meaning or a barrage of demands, of clichéd slogans and shouting. Writer's block is a debasement *by* words which the writer, the servant of words, cannot refute but by an impossibly autocratic act of favouritism that, now outdated, appears mechanical as well as infantile ('the cat sat on the mat'), or else autocracy self-administered as exile ('no work today'; a banishment from the world of words, and from the world of work, as useless as a night spent in the failed pursuit of sleeping).

This anxiety concerning the relative worth of words, as though words were really magical and could wreak havoc in the worlds of their users, is inseparable from the experience of writer's pain we inherit from the Romantic period in the concept of the sublime, the physical limit point and simultaneous occasion of divine inspiration.[2] In her absorbing study *Reading, Writing, and Romanticism: The Anxiety of Reception*, Lucy Newlyn shows how Romantic poets such as Wordsworth and Coleridge invoke the sublime or irreducibly grand qualities of landscape in order to capture in advance the loss that follows on the reader's consumption of the literary work, and convert it to their own writer's ends. If this is not exactly having your cake and eating it, it is close to having your destination before the journey, itself close to the mindset that seems best-suited to ready sleeping, that asks not where we are going at night and what will happen on the way but only at what time we will be returning, as though sleep were not a work in progress but a given.

And yet the sublime, like sleep, by definition that which overwhelms, teeters on the abyss that threatens the mortal claimant to absolute authority absolutely, rather as the rise of print culture, albeit in a much less striking way, expands the author's reach on the condition that it also relativises and dilutes it. Thus, Newlyn claims,

> it might be said [...] that the authoritative voice of Wordworth's criticism masks a deep uncertainty about the direction in which he wishes to move his theory of interpretation – towards the hermeticism on which he over-insists, or towards the hermeneutics of collaboration which implicitly contradicts it [...]. Figures such as the 'gentle maid' in 'Nutting', Dorothy in 'Tintern Abbey', and the traveller in the 'Cave of Yordas' similarly provide reassurance that books are by no means 'exposed and lifeless' after

2 Gerald L. Bruns describes Blanchot as 'one of the last romantics, where romanticism is a name for the persistence of whatever is irreducible or excessive with respect to the Enlightenment's unfinished project of housing everything in its condominium [...]. Poetry is the Enlightenment's "other night", not the Dark Age that it supersedes but that which accompanies it and keeps it awake' (xv). See also Shaviro (110–70); Clark (*Derrida* 64–70).

> publication, but are subject to a vivid continuing life in their readers' minds. The author dies, perhaps – but only perhaps, because a 'new quickening' soon succeeds. (133)

In its necessary dialogue with the emergent phenomenon of mass print availability, the logical correlative of the decline in aristocratic patronage that both frees and daunts the writer, Romanticism bespeaks an ambivalence about the crowd and its relation to the relatively new development of private reading. Discourse on the sublime marks the point of transition from an age in which the production of literature is authorised by a mimetic faithfulness to classical models, to one in which an experience of the failure of mimesis, or the self-sundering of the sublime encounter with nature paradoxically authorises the artist. The artist's new authority arises, in part, from an encounter with his limitations in an experience of painful abasement before wild nature, which is also beginning to be characterised as the realm of lost innocence and thus as an artistic remedy for the unruly exigencies or Revolutionary wildness of the crowd.

The sublime imperils even as it sustains the poet, 'challeng-[ing] the mind's capacity to organize experience', and, in doing so, expanding of necessity the mind (Goldman 176). Yet the pleasurable pain that attends self-extension retains its annihilating promise: sublime experience is moving, and in the attempt to accommodate its moving qualities, the mind itself must be perpetually mobile, even, arguably, homeless. The connection between sublime inspiration and sleeplessness, a mode of destitution which is beginning to glimpse its surplus value without foregoing property rights to mainstream or readerly subjectivity altogether, is strengthened here. But the pain of sublime inspiration can just as readily turn to self-doubt or self-replacement, as it does in the profoundly unhomely genre of the Gothic novel, whose task is to terrify and expand the appetite for painful experience of its readers.

In Edgar Allan Poe's 1840 story 'The Man of the Crowd', the wakeful narrator follows an insomniac in the person of an old man whose fear of solitude causes him to feed on the manic energy generated by the crowd. In his observation of the mass of people passing before the window of a certain Coffee House in London, the narrator discerns, at first, merely a 'tumultuous sea' of persons which quickly separates itself into distinct classes and types in which the narrator himself is not included. In this respect, he is apart from the crowd, but his double is the old man who is already engaged in the act of crowd-watching in a much more desperate and frenetic manner (Poe in Messer 203). The narrator's initial sighting of this figure has painfully sublime or Gothic overtones. His attention is arrested by 'the absolute idiosyncrasy of [the man's] expression' (207) and:

> As I endeavoured, during the brief minute of my original survey, to form some analysis of the meaning conveyed, there arose confusedly and paradoxically within my mind, the idea of vast mental power, of caution, of penuriousness, of avarice, of coolness, of malice, of blood-thirstiness, of triumph, of merriment, of excessive terror, of intense – of extreme despair. I felt singularly aroused, startled, fascinated. 'How wild a history', I said to myself, 'is written within that bosom!' Then came a craving desire to keep the man in view – to know more of him. (207)

The restless old man embodies the fractious energies of the crowd itself as well as its extremes of class and status. Though feeble and thin, his clothes are 'of beautiful texture', and hidden within them the narrator catches a glimpse 'both of a diamond and a dagger' (207). When the crowd thins, he becomes lost and hesitant, but on emerging into the throng of a busy bazaar becomes himself again, entering 'shop after shop, pric[ing] nothing' and not speaking but looking 'at all objects with a wild and vacant stare' (209). Pursuing this eccentric character in 'the wildest amazement' throughout the night, the narrator, although gripped by 'an interest all-absorbing', eventually tires and, at last, gazes fully into the face of the wanderer (210–11). But the old man fails to notice the narrator at all, which leads the narrator to impute to him the 'type and the genius of deep crime. He refuses to be alone. *He is the man of the crowd*' (211). As Ernest Fontana notes:

> The Man of the Crowd resists th[e] natural tendency of the crowd to disassemble and individuate itself through sleep. By remaining awake, he becomes a freakishly unique external man, his unsuspected waking consciousness fully absorbed by the public, exterior life of the London streets. His insomnia thus becomes for Poe emblematic of humanity deprived of individual subjectivity by the conditions of mass urban aggregation, or in terms of Poe's opening metaphor, the insomniac is a text that cannot be read, a text that remains a surface without depth or inwardness. (39)

The irony, of course, is that the narrator is also gripped by the contagious mesmerism of crime's deep genius, its feasting on the presence of a crowd whose internal variety it does not see. And, although eventually falling prey to the humanising influence of the need to sleep, the narrator has equally mesmerised his audience who, perhaps as a result, may be expected to pass a troubled night.

The story's effect lies in the way it conveys the simultaneous threat and power of mass movement, so that the reader, like the speaker, is swept along, our ability to recognise class distinctions operative within the mass notwithstanding. Insomnia, here, plays an interestingly ambiguous role. While aligned with the teeming streets which never sleep, as Fontana claims, the old man himself does not seem to suffer as long as a new crowd can be found. It is the narrator and, by implication, the reader, who suffers from the recognition that there exists such a thing as a crowd demon, an invisible incubus in the form of a mindless man. Given that narrator and reader are at this point at the end of a wakeful night and the implied disruption of a restful one respectively, the association between sleeplessness and mass depravity is somewhat compromised. The Romantic artist is a man apart, who loves his pain, the prototype of the eternal wanderer and the inspired as sleepless meets the man of the crowd, and the reader, in the age of the Gothic novel. If the old man is nothing more than the anarchic spirit of the crowd and the concentration of its teeming qualities, might the Romantic or Gothic writer himself, entranced by this same spirit, be little more than mass culture's contract with the sublime in its continued dissipation of desiring energies?

The answer to this question must turn on the nature of the contract, if that is the right word for it, that the sleepless writer makes with night. I suggest that the insomniac writer, like the wakeful lover, is secretly in love with night, according to that logic by which inspiration, amorous or artistic, can only arrive unsought, and on arrival becomes proof of the perfect reciprocity of its nature, refusing the commonsensical clarity and reductiveness of the day, withdrawing into perpetual secrecy. My lover sees in me what I can't see in myself, what I am blind to, as I in her, as my writing transforms a privacy of pain into a work of art or art's apprentice, in which others find solace or another pain, and as sleep conveys me to the realm in which another writing, and (for the believer at least) another love, operate at a further turn from the illusion of communion allowed by day. In this way, as Blanchot, for instance, holds, a measure of night's surplus energy, which thrives on the absence to itself with which it is credited, so that it escapes the obsessional accounting of the day, is borrowed by writing, on the condition that it can never be credited to the writer him- or herself but resides in the ongoing life of the work, whether as the book that departs, or the writing that continues for another day, another night, a lifetime.

The dream of nirvana habitually withholds itself, that is its nature, whether in the field of love, or of literature (the completed work of art which is yet mine, the perfect reader) or sleeping; the human instance of each – the lover, the writer, the sleeper – is the element that brings it down to earth. A good night's sleep will flee the zealous seeker and is, by definition, sullied and diminished by chemical manipulation, it is love found by advertising (a dirty secret), or writing by the (rule)book, second best. Sleep's guile, like that of love, is really innocence. Blind to itself, it can only ever resist the well laid plan. Sleep, love and writing are masters of exception, and thus servants of daytime's law, but it is only by yielding to their exceptionally unclear workings that such unthought laws as day and night, rules and writing, love as destiny, can be crossed and reconfigured, or arguably, experienced or accorded meaning at all.

On love of pain, the night train, and not stopping writing

> Ah a nice mess we're in the whole pack of us, is it possible we're all in the same boat, no, we're in a nice mess each one in his own peculiar way.
>
> Samuel Beckett, *The Unnamable* (372).

In claiming that the insomniac writer is in love with night, I want to emphasise the constructive role of night's, and sleep's secrecy. Insomnia is not so much the impossibility of sleep as sleep's delay; thus the sufferer is not shut out of the communication circuit as with other, more taxing kinds of pain – for instance, the sufferer whose physical pain eats up the chance of sleep as it does all other respite, harrowing language so that language is all trauma, nothing but a relentless gape and rend, the world as pain. The challenge the insomniac faces is not one of self-extinction but of waiting, and the question of how to wait, in so far as the quality of one's waiting for sleep has a direct, but impossible to guess at, relation to the likelihood of sleep's arrival.

The insomniac's task arises from the indiscernible nature of sleep's contract with the day: we don't know when the sleep train will arrive because we haven't the body-as-organism's perspective on the costs of the endeavours of the daytime journey, we have only consciousness, on whose extinction sleep depends. This makes the work, if such it can be called, of waiting for sleep like that of courting love, or labouring at authorial inspiration, perfect contradictions of the kind that, seeming to flirt with fate, yet annul, and in a sense protect it as ideal through opposition, at the same time refusing its unknowable temporality, its arrival's incipient surprise. By refusing to wait, the would-be sleeper or lover or writer keeps faith with the exclusion of the state that she subtends. Sleeplessness, I have come to think, is incurably romantic to the extent that romance can only tell the saleable elements of love, its sublime landscape of peaks and troughs, the substance of the reader's diminishing return. What the romance of the sleepless writer cannot tell is the tale of sleep's desire, for which we need another kind of logic, an unconscious logic or a logic of the journey, whose lease on the daytime world is mortgaged on the strength of night's ability to pose and re-pose any day's given questions. Night's task is to practise this hidden labour and to converse, in its own language, with the body's habitation of mortality as limit and as pain.

What is it in us that loves our pain, that suffers, enjoyably, at the expense of the self, as love and writing seem to require that we do? That those who do not sleep and who write and go on not sleeping, fear that sleeping in an ordinary way will diminish creative power, are onto something I am sure, but what kind of something this is I remain uncertain. Hirsch is proud of the poverty of sleeplessness. 'Everyone has a share of the dream kingdom', he writes,

> but mine is a minor one. There are writers who build huge gothic mansions in the rolling countryside of sleep, but I merely lease a room in someone else's apartment building crouched by the side of a busy road. All night trucks lumber by and the ground rumbles underfoot. I own nothing here. (58)

The poverty of the night worker is indistinguishable from riches, as the line between sleep and dreams has been commandeered for poetry, or something greater: 'the black hole of four A.M. [...] the hour with its head in its hands' (61). Hirsch even describes poetry as his 'purchase on the night kingdom [...] a kind of payment to eternity for the lifelong gift of sleeplessness' (63), a hopeful domestication or diminishment of death. I am not convinced by this.

In 'Literature as Symptom', Colette Soler offers the Lacanian understanding of symptom as desire's invention, its form of being in the world which is the history of its living in each body, as a work of reading, and, by extension, writing. 'What does it mean to create?' she asks:

> The answer is: to bring something into being where there was nothing before. But saying 'where there was nothing', I already imply a place. And there is no such thing as a place without the symbolic and its marks, and every symbolic mark engenders as empty the place that it creates. (215)

It is this kind of emptiness that sleep, and love, and writing also engender, an emptiness which must not be understood, prematurely, as the cowed object of jurisdiction, as so many readers of the early Lacan still insist, but the enfleshed exception that gives meaning to the law on the condition that it cannot be included specifically within it. As Copjec explains, 'the subject is never fully determinate according to psychoanalysis, which treats this indeterminateness as a real feature of the subject', as opposed to the historicist approach which gives indeterminacy a false value, so that it tends to revert to the sum total of contingencies of a culture or an era, a confidence trick, democracy's guile, *plus ça change* [...] and so on:

> The historicist response to psychoanalysis approaches the universal subject as a vague concept that can, with more or less effort and a better knowledge of history, be given more precise attributes. This hasty historicism fails to understand that the universal subject is not a *vague* concept but, in Charles S. Peirce's sense of the term, a *general* one. That is, the concept does not poorly or wrongly describe a subject whose structure is actually determinate but precisely indicates a subject that is in some sense *objectively indeterminate*. Against the faddish critique of the universal subject, psychoanalysis insists on this concept's political importance. (*Read* 147)

As Copjec goes on to note, the indeterminate nature of the subject, in psychoanalytic terms, is strictly relational: the ego, or the Cartesian subject of mythical self-sufficiency, is nothing more, and nothing less, than the subject as lost object – the claim I make to expressive validity in the already existing world of words, the temporary lease I hold on silence or the night – under the sign of love, where love is the giving of an indeterminacy one does not know one has, in the guise of the image of perfect communion (147–8). Or in other words, love is blind, and it is through the specific blindness of love to its own workings, as of sleep to night, that love makes meaning, that in the guise of recognition in the eyes of another I am reconciled to the object status of myself.[3]

This is why Lacan says that 'all love, subsisting only on the basis of the "stops not being written"', that is, operational thanks to a negation, as love is something more than friendship, and something else than pain, and is unable to be summoned, or bought, or earned, and persists in the shape of a future as yet unknown, or a lover who retains the power to wound, or to leave me, 'tends to make the negation shift to the "doesn't stop being written", doesn't stop, won't stop' (145). If it were really ceaseless, that is, went on forever, love could not work, any more than sleep can work, so far as we know, once it is the final sleep, or than writing can work once it is fully present to the writer. The perfect piece of writing I make will be my last, as will the perfect sleep, for there will be no more intrigue between myself and writing after that, nor between myself and sleeping either. Or, as is fortunately more likely, I will find in the morning that the words written yesterday are like last night's dishes or last night's

3 In her latest book Copjec clarifies the Lacanian position of *Seminar XI*: 'When one loves something, one loves something in it that is more than itself, its nonidentity to itself. But a new point can be made […]. To say that what we love in the object is something more than that object is not to say only that we love that real point in the object from where it can cease being what it was to become something different from itself', which we might gloss as love's possibility or love's high vision, 'but also that *what we love in the object is the object in ourselves*', our contingency (79). 'One must refrain from the temptation to turn this observation back into a banality by making it a matter of resemblance; one does not find in the loved object a reflection of one's own image […] one finds rather in the jouissance loving it affords a corporeal experience of the self […]. The lover […] is locatable only in the object, the partial object or indivisible remainder of the act of love. Indivisible (because irreducible to spatiotemporal coordinates) *and* the product of no division, part of no whole' (79–80).

dreams, and, after doing or recounting, will take a day's to- and fro-ing in the happy sullying, forgetting and doing of again.

Long time waiting

> The palms do not sing,
> nor does the breast.
> What sings is what says silent.
>
> Adam Zagajewski, 'Where the Breath Is' (22).

> In insomnia it is the night itself that watches. It watches.
>
> Emmanuel Lévinas, *Existence and Existents* (66).

In love, the subject surrenders what it *lacks* to the Other – to language, and to others in so far as common language bars their way, and thwarts love as communion – on condition that the Other continue to uphold the lack-in-being that is desire. To love is to bank on one's vulnerability, to give an ideally lifelong value to waiting and unknowing, where one's desire is aimed at the particular absolute, as Copjec calls it, or the unique unknowability in which love consists, the movement of the self-vacating of the beloved's desire, the way s/he loves, the style of his or her embodying of love's emptiness in the interests of its gain (Copjec 148–9; also Berlant 2001). Love, like sleep and writing, is formally beautiful, which is why it can only be cheapened by guarantee. It already contains its guarantee in the form of mortal yielding, a reenactment of the ordeal between the human being as organism – governed by the energetic wrangling of the drives – and linguistic mediation which catches up the body and lends it a productive absence that it can never close while living, a gap to reach across, a sleep of reason that the sleeping body borrows back: love's good fortune, fortune's guile.

Sleeping, like loving and writing, can be practised but all the work is nought if there is not, at some point, a falling away from work, a surrender or at the very least a slip up, a falling in. So it is that in a perfect dream, I have only to chance a footstep into the frame of my heart's desire to be found alone and waking, my waking self the instance of the missed perfection's making. In all its forms the dream of oneness, whether of the perfect reader, of writer's value as fullness, of sleep as that which both restores me to myself and yet will come when I call, miraculous provider, needs a trick to work, does not stop not being written, as Lacan says of the work of the unconscious in the land of dreaming (144).

What Lacan figures enigmatically here, in the famously difficult seminar on love and finitude, is the way the bid for love, and by extension in the reading I am proposing, sleep and the work of art, arises from the place in the social field that marks the instance of my own uniqueness, which can never be positively claimed. To the extent that it is claimed, in Lacanian terms, the living history of my desire or uniqueness appears as symptom or *sinthome*, the not being quite at home with oneself that makes desiring subjectivity work, and gives it an imaginary substance and a real, embodied history, lived as a gap between a subject and the objects of her desire. Laying claim to my own *sinthome*, however, blinds me to my desire, in the sense that when I say 'I have trouble sleeping', I identify with trouble, refusing knowledge of what I gain by trouble's intervention. I cannot identify with trouble and at the same time reach the sleep that I desire, just as I cannot know love without a corresponding ignorance. At the moment I see what my lover sees in me, we are both diminished; love is ailing, or has died.

The empty place offered to the subject by language is a place I encompass without ever getting close to it, a source that I embody without mastery and that persists in my writing and my speaking as the relation I have to my own death, my eventual demise in sleep, the end of love and writing in insufferable communion (see Ragland 84–114; Copjec 259–60; Verhaeghe 137).[4] It makes my writing and my sleeping a foreign body that yet functions as the irreducible instance of who I am, rather than of who I would like to think I am, which is endlessly reducible and, by turns, prone to imaginative expanding (as W.G. Sebald says of Stendhal's, alias Henri Beyle's, decision to vacate Napoleon's fallen army, in a phrase which would make many a youthfully ambitious author blush: 'At all events, it was in the autumn that he resolved to become the greatest writer of all time' (18)).

And this bizarre reverse specificity of sleep, love, and writing is why, as Blanchot says, I can never find myself in my own writing as other than love's idiot, playing with clothes made for grown-ups, or else in the assumption of clear competence as disguise, and why I cannot ever know whether it is sleeping or lying awake that inclines me toward writing, and to which state writing bears the strongest likeness or productive claim. And therefore whether writing arises in the bliss of imaginative completion, as when I wake after eight or nine hours fortunate furlough in the land of dreams to fall, hope renewed, onto the keyboard, or the hermetic ordeal of sleeplessness as ersatz pain: a head start, a working superstition, a stutter at infinity, a trial round.

This may be, in the end, the tenor of the painfulness that connects insomnia and writing, the perpetually anxious, but at the same time saving supplement of the *cannot know*, what Lévinas seems to invoke when he claims that in insomnia, one exists as 'the object rather than the subject of an anonymous thought' (66).

4 J.-B. Pontalis, although not Lacanian, provides a sense of the subject as lost object in his richly evocative clinical writings on pain. For instance: 'Where there is pain, it is the absent, lost object that is present; it is the actual, present object that is absent. Consequently the pain of separation appears to be secondary to a naked, absolute pain.' [Pontalis notes here that 'this is perhaps what Lacan had in mind when one day he referred to "*la douleur d'exister*"']. The psychic scene is populated only by shadows, the psychic *reality* is elsewhere, not so much repressed as encysted' (Pontalis 200, 211n).

Not a thought without a thinker, but the residue of a thought, the mortal remains, transience as the work of breath and life, something to be going on with. For the habitually sleepless, Hamlet's question does not need asking before the night becomes too full of guile and fraught with actorly waking, whether a comic or a tragic occasion is moot. Sleeplessness is the existentialist's nemesis *par excellence*, which probably makes it a tragicomedy if not farce. It simply doesn't matter whether you choose or refuse it; it already has your number and the mode of your refusal, it knows something you don't about the ends of dreams, something you can't not want to know, something about the work of writing as thankful self-vacation, about love as the faint true heart of fiction, about the world before you were in it, up all night, making trouble. It knows something about waking and something about madness, as Muriel Rukeyser says, and, as a rehearsal for the exile that is not like love and writing but grants them a measure of its mythic charge, its secret history, something about your going that you can only practise while you're waiting, listening for the warning horn from just around the corner, heralding oblivion, hoping for the best.

Works Cited

Beckett, Samuel. *Three Novels: Molloy; Malone Dies; The Unnamable.* Trans. Patrick Bowles. New York: Grove P, 1958.

Berlant, Lauren. "Love, a Queer Feeling." *Homosexuality and Psychoanalysis.* Ed. Tim Dean and Christopher Lane. Chicago & London: U of Chicago P, 2001. 432–51.

Blanchot, Maurice. *The Space of Literature.* Trans. Ann Smock. Lincoln, Nebraska & London: U of Nebraska P, 1982.

— "From Dread to Language." *The Station Hill Blanchot Reader.* Trans. Lydia Davis *et al.* Barrytown, New York: Station Hill, 1999. 343–58.

Bruns, Gerald L. *Maurice Blanchot: The Refusal of Philosophy.* Baltimore & London: Johns Hopkins UP, 1997.

Clark, Timothy. 1992. *Derrida, Heidegger, Blanchot: Sources of Derrida's Notion and Practice of Literature.* Cambridge: CUP, 1992.
— 1997. *The Theory of Inspiration: Composition as a Crisis of Subjectivity in Romantic and Post-Romantic Writing.* Manchester and New York: Manchester UP, 1997.
Connor, Steven. *Dumbstruck: A Cultural History of Ventriloquism.* Oxford: OUP, 2000.
Copjec, Joan. "The Subject Defined by Suffrage." *Lacanian ink* 7 (1993): 47–58.
— *Read My Desire: Lacan Against the Historicists.* Cambridge, Mass., & London: MIT Press, 1994.
— "The Tomb of Perseverance: On *Antigone*." *Giving Ground: The Politics of Propinquity.* Ed. Joan Copjec and Michael Sorkin. London & New York: Verso, 1999. 233–66.
— *Imagine There's No Woman: Ethics and Sublimation.* Cambridge, Mass., & London: MIT P, 2002.
Deagon, Andrea. "The Twelve Hours of Night: Insomnia and Transformation in *Gilgamesh*." *Soundings* 81. 3/4 (Fall/Winter 1998): 461–89.
Fontana, Ernest. "Literary Insomnia." *New Orleans Review* 17. 2 (Summer 1990): 38–42.
Goldman, Marlene. *Paths of Desire: Images of Exploration and Mapping in Canadian Women's Writing.* Toronto: U of Toronto P, 1997.
Hirsch, Edward. "Sleeplessness." *Night Errands: How Poets Use Dreams.* Ed. Rod Townley. Pittsburgh: U of Pittsburgh P, 1998. 58–63.
Kafka, Franz. *Gesammelte Werke in zwölf Bänden.* Ed. Hans-Gerd Koch. Frankfurt am Mainz: Fischer. Vol. 3, *Der Proces*, 1994.
Lacan, Jacques. 1998. *The Seminar of Jacques Lacan, Book XX: On Feminine Sexuality, the Limits of Love and Knowledge.* Trans. Bruce Fink. New York: W.W. Norton and Co, 1998.
Lévinas, Emmanuel. *Existence and Existents.* Trans. Alphonso Lingis. Dordrecht: Kluwer Academic Publishers, 1988.
Messer, Jane. Introduction. *Bedlam: An Anthology of Sleepless Nights.* Ed. Jane Messer. Sydney: Allen and Unwin, 1996. xiv–xx.
Miller, Jacques-Alain. "*Extimité*." *Prose Studies* 11. 3 (1988): 121–30.
Newlyn, Lucy. *Reading, Writing, and Romanticism: The Anxiety of Reception.* Oxford: OUP, 2000.
Poe, Edgar Allan. "The Man of the Crowd." *Bedlam: An Anthology of Sleepless Nights.* Ed. Jane Messer. Sydney: Allen and Unwin, 1996. 202–11.
Pontalis, J.-B. *Frontiers in Psychoanalysis: Between the Dream and Psychic Pain.* Trans. Catherine Cullen & Philip Cullen. London: Hogarth P and the Institute for Psycho-Analysis, 1981.
Ragland, Ellie. 1995. *Essays on the Pleasures of Death from Freud to Lacan.* New York & London: Routledge, 1995.

Rilke, Rainer Maria. *The Notebooks of Malte Laudrides Brigge.* Trans. M.D. Herder Norton. *Bedlam: An Anthology of Sleepless Nights.* Ed. Jane Messer. Sydney: Allen and Unwin, 1996. 284–5.

Scarry, Elaine. *The Body in Pain: The Making and Unmaking of the World.* Oxford and New York: OUP, 1985.

Schweizer, Harold. "Against Suffering: A Meditation on Literature." *Literature and Medicine* 19. 2 (2000): 229–40.

Sebald, W.G. *Vertigo.* Trans. Michael Hulse. London: Vintage, 1999.

Shaviro, Steven. *Passion and Excess: Blanchot, Bataille, and Literary Theory.* Tallahassee: Florida State UP, 1990.

Soler, Colette. "Literature as Symptom." *Lacan and the Subject of Language.* Ed. Ellie Ragland-Sullivan & Mark Bracher. New York and London: Routledge, 1991. 213–19.

Spaar, Lisa Russ. "To *Sleep*, Perchance: The Poetry of Insomnia." *Chronicle of Higher Education* 47. 9 (2000): B12–13.

Thomson, James. "*'City of Dreadful Night' and Other Poems.*" London: Bertram Dobell, 1910.

Verhaeghe, Paul. "Lacan's Answer to the Classical Mind/Body Deadlock: Retracing Freud's *Beyond.*" *Reading Seminar XX: Lacan's Major Work on Love, Knowledge, and Feminine Sexuality.* Ed. Suzanne Barnard & Bruce Fink. Albany, New York: S.U.N.Y P, 2002. 109–39.

Zagajewski, Adam. *Without End: New and Selected Poems.* Trans. Clare Cavanagh *et al.* New York: Farrar, Straus and Giroux, 2002.

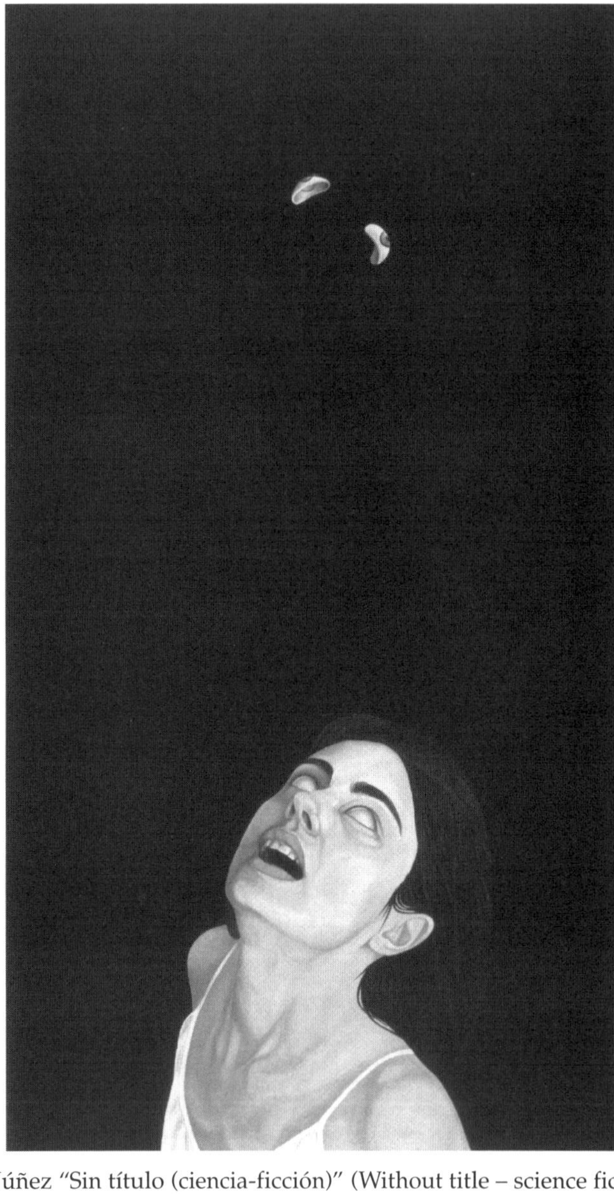

Marina Núñez "Sin título (ciencia-ficción)" (Without title – science fiction). Private Collection, Barcelona, 1998.

Under the Aspect of Pain

Kerstin Bergman
Lund University

One of the most intricate investigations of pain in Swedish literature is found in the novel *Death of a Beekeeper* from 1978. This is one of Lars Gustafsson's most philosophically interesting, not to mention very well-known, novels. The protagonist, Lars Lennart Westin, is approaching 40 and dying from spleen cancer. He spends the last year of his life alone in an isolated countryside house in Sweden, writing down thoughts, observations, memories and experiences in three notebooks: The Yellow Book, in which he mainly writes things concerning his everyday life, the Blue Book where fantasy, fiction and imaginative thoughts dominate, and the Damaged Book – which is really more of a phone pad – where things concerning communication can be found. Central in all of the notebooks, as well as in Westin's life during his last months, is the pain caused by his tumor. Most of his thoughts are inspired by, or directly reflect, the experience of pain. The notes, found after Westin's death, reconstruct his world as they are left to speak for themselves, and the only way to access his life and pain is thus as mediated by language. But what knowledge is there to be gained from Westin's experiences?

As it turns out, pain has important implications on many different levels of the novel. To a great extent, *Death of a Beekeeper* is a novel about the possibilities and limitations of language. Between the lines, although never explicitly mentioned, hovers the spirit of Ludwig Wittgenstein. Not only does Westin have many biographical details in common with the Cambridge philosopher, but also the majority of the examples he uses in discussing language in his notebooks are borrowed from Wittgenstein, most notably from his *Philosophische Untersuchungen/Philosophical Investigations*.

Westin ponders why language has not developed words for distinguishing different kinds of pain, when it has words that can be used to describe different shades of color, for example, in a very detailed way. His conclusion is that: 'Perhaps that is because two people can see the same colors while two people can not possibly experience the same pain?' (22).[1] The underlying idea is Wittgenstein's private language argument. In discussing this, Wittgenstein himself also uses pain as the example. The main point of the argument, which has been subject to extensive criticism, is that the development of language is based upon common experiences. Therefore, a language can never be developed for the things people cannot share, which implies that there can never be such a thing as a private language.

Also, in the philosophical and theoretical literature on pain, the limitations of language are often in focus. Harvard scholar Elaine Scarry stresses, in her book *The Body in Pain* that pain's 'resistance to language is not simply one of its incidental or accidental attributes but it is essential to what it is' (5). This is a statement that is well in line with Wittgenstein's private language argument, and it also expresses something crucial about pain.

The difficulty of expressing pain through words is not an issue occupying only philosophers; it has long been a problem within the medical community as well. Many attempts have been made to work around it by creating an appropriate terminology. In 1973, Ronald Melzack and W.S. Torgerson developed the so-called 'McGill Pain Questionnaire' which has been widely used in hospitals and pain clinics ever since.[2] They collected the words most often spoken by patients or used in articles on pain, and arranged those words into different categories (*Challenge* 38). These word groups are then shown to patients suffering from

1 'Kanske är det för att två människor kan se samma färg, men två människor omöjligt kan känna samma smärta?' (*Biodlaren* 39–40).

2 The questionnaire was first presented in Ronald Melzack's *The Puzzle of Pain* (New York: Basic, 1973), and then in a revised edition co-authored by Patrick D. Wall called *The Challenge of Pain* (New York: Basic, 1983).

pain to help them describe what they are feeling without having to create a 'private language' to do so. The McGill questionnaire seems to have provided a breakthrough in allowing patients to describe their experiences. According to people administering it, avoiding the difficulty of coming up with your own words of description provides a great relief to many patients in pain.

In Gustafsson's novel, Westin refuses to accept any confirmation of the fact that he is terminally ill. He avoids any contact with the hospital and refuses to open the letters they send him, so he never becomes aware of this clinical terminology. Westin still does not give up his attempts to put his private experience into words. In one of his more successful attempts, he seems pretty convincing:

> Right now, for example, I feel a pulsing pain, which in a few minutes is going to keep me from finishing these sentences. It begins pretty far down somewhere in the right calf, where it feels something like liquid metal, or like something which has hooked into the musculature, a golden wire one could perhaps say. Then it radiates to the right loin, sends, along the back of the leg, a whole bundle of white radiating gold wires to the navel and the hip, and a fan of this radiating gold extends up to the diaphragm. When I lie down, it hurts twice as much; when I remain seated, it wanders up to the back, it doesn't always maintain the same pitch, the frequencies, the decibel count of the white radiating gold changes constantly, they create chords, very clean, clear chords, until they suddenly get tangled somehow and become *cutting*. (69–70)[3]

3 'Just nu känner jag till exempel en pulserande smärta som inom några minuter kommer att hindra mig från att skriva det här till slut. Den börjar en bra bit ner på höger lår, där den känns ungefär som om en flytande metall eller något sådant hade trasslat in sig i muskulaturen, en gyllene tråd skulle man kanske kunna säga. Sedan fortsätter den upp mot högra ljumsken, skickar ut hela knippen av vitlysande guldtrådar ända upp mot naveln ut mot höften, mot benets baksida, det ligger en solfjäder av dova ekon av det där lysande guldet upp mot mellangärdet. Om jag lägger mig ner gör det dubbelt så ont; om jag fortsätter sitta sprider det sig upp mot ryggen, det håller inte hela tiden samma ton, frekvenserna, svängningstalen i det där vitlysande guldet skiftar hela tiden, det bildar ackord, riktigt snygga ackord tills de går i baklås på något sätt och blir *skärande*' (*Biodlaren* 108–109).

Westin's account is sublime in its fusing of beautiful images and crass reality. His description falls under what Melzack and Torgerson refers to as the '*sensory qualities*' of pain. In the McGill questionnaire, these include groups of words describing 'temporal, spatial, pressure, thermal and other properties' of pain (*Challenge* 38).[4]

It is interesting to note that the metaphors chosen by Westin to describe his inner experience are mainly taken from the areas of 'outer' sensory experience. He uses visually perceptible patterns like wires, bundles and fans, and color-related words and phrases like golden and 'white radiating'. He also uses things you can hear, such as pitches, frequencies, decibel count and chords.[5]

In describing his pain, Westin tries to overcome the limitations of language, but as the quote illustrates, and as he actually explicitly states there, even if he finds words, they are only applicable up to a certain point. When pain becomes too intense, or, in Westin's words, when the chords 'get tangled somehow and become *cutting*' (70), he is unable to continue describing the pain. He cannot even put this stage of pain into words after the pain has passed.

4 In addition to *sensory qualities*, they suggest that pain can also be described in terms of *affective qualities*, and by *evaluative* or cognitive words (*Challenge* 38).

5 In addition to these metaphors from the areas of *vision* and *hearing*, he adds the area of *touch*, when he uses the image of the sun, and thereby creates a strong sense of heat: 'A terrible, unheard of, white hot, impersonal power is taking its residence in my nervous system, occupies it to the last molecule and tries to explode every nerve into a cloud of blinding white gases, as in the corona of the sun (the whole night I thought about sun protuberances, the way they pulse, the way they break forth in cascades on the surface of the sun)' (*Beekeeper* 79). 'En fruktansvärd, oerhörd, vidglödgad, opersonlig kraft [som] slår sig ner i mitt nervsystem, ockuperar det till den sista molekylen och försöker spränga varje nerv till ett moln av vitglödgande gaser, som i – i solkoronan (jag tänkte hela natten på solprotuberanser, hur de pulserar, hur de slår upp som kaskader över solytan)' (*Biodlaren* 121–2).

Elaine Scarry states that to 'witness the moment when pain causes a reversion to the pre-language of cries and groans is to witness the destruction of language' (6). In a paradoxical way, Westin here enacts that moment by way of narration through his use of language. We, as readers, cannot hear his cries and groans, but instead we witness how his notes become more and more fragmented until he grows completely silent and the page turns blank. After one such an episode, the next chapter begins with a short comment from the editor of Westin's notes: '(no notes whatsoever for thirty-three days)', and then Westin himself continues: 'April 6th. The pains are beginning to go away. Now only emptiness' (101).[6] The editor's comment and the short, fragmented sentences used by Westin indicate something of what he has been going through, but it also enforces the fact that his pain has been beyond the reach of language. This is an effective way of thus illustrating the destruction of language described by Scarry.

But, in *Death of a Beekeeper* pain does not only show the limitations of language. It has a productive aspect as well, in that it functions as a means for Westin to reach beyond the surface of language in order to experience something more real and original. At one point, he even claims that the last months of pain have made him real (152). Throughout the novel, and thanks to his pain, Westin works his way down, or back, to something basic. The structure is clearly detectable in the chapter headlines where it can be seen how he writes his way through his marriage, his childhood, further past God, and finally through paradise.

Westin notes that the pain is altering his priorities. The ages and memories that now seem important to him are not prioritized as before. The memories of marriage and working life mean nothing anymore. Instead, his childhood now seems to be the

6 In the Swedish original, Westin's words are even more fragmented than in the English translation: '[...] (under trettiotre dagar över huvud taget inga anteckningar) Den 6 april. Smärtorna avtar. Bara en tomhet' (153).

only really important part of his life. He suggests 'perhaps pain is making me lonely again and egocentric like a child' (63).[7]

The experience of pain successively increases the distance between Westin and the rest of the world. It's almost like he enters into a world of his own. The only other human beings whose company he enjoys during the months related in the novel are two young boys from the neighborhood. He finds that he can relate to them because they remind him of himself. Perhaps this is because when Westin reaches beyond language, he reaches a state similar to that of a child who has not yet completely conquered language. Without language the child, as well as Westin, can be considered being closer to the real, unmediated world and maybe also to a more spiritual side of reality.

For the longest time, Westin felt secure in the idea that the pain was his and only his. It reduced his desire to interact with the rest of the world, and allowed him to hide within himself. Eventually, he comes to realize that pain has shown him that 'I have a body, no, that I *am* a body' (78).[8] But, as time passes, the pains are destroying this body and he realizes that the 'foundation of the entire concept of the self is that it will continue to exist tomorrow' (79).[9] If he is his body and that body dies, there is nothing left, or in Westin's words: pain is 'a precise measure of the forces which hold this body together. It is a precise measure of the force which *has made* my existence possible'. (80, my italics).[10] The past tense used here enforces the fact that Westin's 'I' is fading. On several occasions, he talks about how his sense of 'I' is dissolving and how his 'I' is becoming nothing more than a word, which no longer has a reference. The center, where the 'I' used to be, is now empty. As to enforce this, he keeps repeating:

7 '[K]anske är det så att smärtan gör mig ensam och självupptagen på barndomens sätt igen' (99).

8 '[J]ag har en kropp, nej att jag *är* en kropp' (120).

9 'Hela idén om jaget bygger på att det kommer finnas till i morgon också' (123).

10 '[E]tt exakt mått på de krafter som håller den här kroppen samman. Den är ett exakt mått på den kraft som *gjorde att jag kunde* existera' (123, my italics).

'I am a body. Nothing but a body. Everything which has to be done, which can be done, must happen within this body' (103).[11]

David B. Morris presents an interesting theory of internally inflicted pain in his book *The Culture of Pain* from 1991. He proposes that pain to a great extent exists only in our mind. Therefore, it can be viewed as a psychological and cultural product rather than a pure physical reality. According to Morris, it is clear that it is 'the brain, ultimately, that allows us to feel pain' (156). He also notes that pain can be produced even 'in the absence of tissue damage' (157), and that it can persist long after an injury is completely healed or even when there is no body to experience the pain as in the case of phantom limb pain (157–8). He also stresses the fact that the experience of pain has to be a conscious act and that 'nonconscious pain is a contradiction in terms' (158).

Westin's spleen cancer ought to fit into the category of internally inflicted painful experiences included in Morris' study. However, Morris' focus on the role of the mind in the experience of pain is not in accordance with Westin's claim that he is exclusively body. This, in addition to Westin's dismissal of the 'I', makes the concept of pain deducted from the novel incompatible with any theory of pain that focuses on the mind.[12]

A theory more applicable to Westin's account of pain can be found in Elaine Scarry's studies of externally inflicted pain. In her writings on torture, she states that extreme pain wipes out all other inner processes of consciousness. She bases her study on interviews of victims and executors of torture, gathered by Amnesty International. Scarry observes that when subject to extreme pain, the victim's senses stop functioning like windows through which the surrounding world can be perceived. Instead they work

11 'Jag är en kropp. Bara en kropp. Allt som måste göras, som kan göras, måste göras inne i denna kropp' (156).

12 The dismissal of the 'I' becomes stronger as the novel unfolds, and in one of his very last notes, Westin writes: 'I, I, I, I, ... after only four times a senseless word.' (Gustafsson, *Beekeeper* 157) 'Jag, jag, jag, jag, ... efter bara fyra gånger ett meningslöst ord' (229).

like exits, pushing the world out, and screening the individual from his or her surroundings. Scarry talks about pain as being 'world-destroying' (29), which in the context means that, while a victim is subject to extreme pain, the rest of the world ceases to exist for him or her. Everything, except the pain, disappears as if it was extinguished from the face of the earth. The victim is reduced to being just a body in pain.

In addition to the accounts by torture victims and tormenters, Scarry exemplifies her discussion by discussing the experience of Pablo Ibbetia in Jean-Paul Sartre's short story 'Le Mur' from 1939. She quotes Ibbetia's realization that he will die 'soon', and then concludes:

> Whenever death can be assigned as 'soon' the dying has already begun. Ibbetia is dying not because he has yet experienced the damage that will end his life but because he has begun to experience the body that will end his life, the body that can be killed, and which when killed will carry away the conditions that allow him to exist. (31)

This is the state Westin is approaching in the novel. This is clearly illustrated by his identification with his dying body and his definition of pain as 'a precise measure of the forces which hold this body together' (80). However, unlike Ibbetia, Westin is already experiencing the 'damage that will end his life', and he does not regard himself as dying even though that is obvious to the reader. In fact, Westin remains hopeful even in the end when he is waiting for the ambulance that will take him to the hospital.

Throughout the novel, Westin's world is shrinking, becoming smaller and smaller, while his 'I' and his body weaken. Even though his pain is not inflicted from the outside, as in the case of torture, or in Ibbetia's case the forthcoming execution, it is clear that the effect is the same as Scarry describes. And occasionally, Westin actually does describe the tumor as something almost external, like an alien thing that is inflicting his pain and suffering.[13]

13 For example when he describes the tumor as a 'wild animal' (*Beekeeper* 78).

Even though he is hopeful, Westin, like Ibbetia, ponders on death as it is coming closer. He means that 'there is no real escape from life. One can only postpone the decision with cunning and cleverness. But there is no way out. It is a totally closed system, and at the exit there is only death. And that naturally is no exit at all' (103).[14]

Death is often described as a door opening up to an afterlife, but Westin has realized that this is a false image. The door cannot be opened, and behind it, it is just as empty as behind the mysterious door in August Strindberg's *A Dream Play*. After realizing this, Westin repaints the door to his house. In his eyes, it turns into a 'mysterious work of art' (105),[15] and thus into nothing but an artifact; an image of a door created by human hand.

But, if there is nothing beyond death, is there no paradise either? This is an issue to which Westin dedicates a lot of thought. Finally, he reaches the conclusion that paradise is the absence of pain, and thus exists here on earth, in the world perceptible by the senses, in the everyday life. Enthusiastically he exclaims: 'That means, however, that we live in Paradise as long as we have no pain! And we don't even know it' (104).[16] But this worldly paradise is unattainable without the preceding pain: 'When the pains stopped fourteen days ago, that was a return for me into a kind of original paradise. But the precondition for this was the pain. It was a form of truth' (111).[17]

14 '[A]tt det inte finns någon verklig utväg ur livet. Det går bara att skjuta upp avgörandet, med skicklighet och list. Men det finns ingen väg ut. Det är ett fullständigt slutet system, och vid utgången finns bara döden. Och det är naturligtvis ingen utgång alls' (*Biodlaren* 156).

15 '[H]emlighetsfullt konstverk' (159).

16 '[S]å länge vi inte har några smärtor lever vi i Paradiset! Lyckliga och olyckliga lever i samma värld, och de ser det inte!' (158).

17 'När smärtorna [...] upphörde, återställdes ett slags ursprungligt paradis för mig. Men förutsättningen för det var smärtan. Den var en form av sanning [...]. Nu skulle man kunna bygga upp ett slags värden igen' (167).

For Westin, pain functions as a lens that makes him see through the haze of deceiving images and ideas and opens up his eyes to the truth about life and the world. Pain obscures everything minor, until only the most real and important stand out in clear light. The description of the paradisiacal state as being 'original' has a resemblance to Westin's pain causing an upgrade of the importance of his childhood and identification with the two young boys who visit him, as mentioned earlier. The childhood becomes a symbol of the original and real which represents something beyond the illusory habits and beliefs gained through the years spent growing into an adult.

Pain has thus given Westin a new and more positive view of life and the world. Suddenly, he perceives life as blissful and sees new possibilities. He starts questioning the lonely and almost anti-social life he has chosen for himself. After realizing that life is all there is, he thinks he might have been better off leading a more socially active life.

He also comes to the conclusion that he ought to have handled his pain differently. He should have fought it at the social level, with the help of other people at the hospital, instead of making it an exclusively private matter. Westin arrives at this conclusion as a result of experiencing the severe pain, and the sad consequence of his insight is that if he had handled that very pain differently, he could have survived – and found bliss and paradise, in life.

The American philosopher and poet George Santayana once said, 'If pain could have cured us we should long ago have been saved' (224). Westin learns a lot from being in pain. When he finally realizes that there is nothing beyond death, and that bliss and paradise can only be acquired within this world, it's already too late. Even though his last words, written down while waiting for the ambulance that will finally take him to the hospital, is '[o]ne can still hope' (158),[18] it is obvious to the reader that for

18 'Man kan alltid hoppas.' (230)

Westin, there is no longer hope. For him, pain's lesson was a wasted effort. He is already far beyond salvation. For his readers, however, Westin's account constitutes a productive experience that may outline a way to avoid making the same mistakes he made.

Works Cited

Gustafsson, Lars. *En biodlares död*. Stockholm, Swed.: Norstedts, 1978.

— *Death of a Beekeeper*. Trans. Janet K. Swaffar and Guntram H. Weber. New York: New Directions, 1981.

Melzack, Ronald and Wall, Patrick D. *The Challenge of Pain*. 2nd ed. London: Penguin, 1996.

Morris, David B. *The Culture of Pain*. Berkeley: U of California P, 1991.

Santayana, George. *The Life of Reason; or The Phases of Human Progress, vol. 1: Introduction, and Reason in Common Sense*, New York: C. Scribner's Sons, 1905.

Scarry, Elaine. *The Body in Pain: The Making and Unmaking of the World*. New York: Oxford UP, 1985.

III. Contagion through Looking

From Pain to Pleasure: Moral Education through Sublime Terror in *The Mysteries of Udolpho*

Valérie de Courville Nicol
Concordia University

This essay[1] focuses on the influence of Edmund Burke's *A Philosophical Enquiry into the Origin of Our Ideas of the Sublime and the Beautiful* on Ann Radcliffe's gothic novel *The Mysteries of Udolpho*, where the production of 'mental pain' through the mechanisms of sublime terror is posed as useful in achieving moral conduct and social order. In conclusion it is argued that gothic subjectivity provides important clues on the role of fear in modern self-government. Its relation to the constitution of feminine bourgeois subjectivity is briefly explored.

The governmental strategies developed by Burke and Radcliffe can be situated in the call for discipline and more humane forms of punishment from the seventeenth century onwards. As Michel Foucault has shown, the humanisation of punishment is conditioned by the imperative of increasing the efficacy of governmental control in light of the unpredictable effects of arbitrary modes of power. Foucault argues that the humanist penal reforms implemented at the turn of the nineteenth century are part of an important shift in the exercise of power. As power moves inwards, it increasingly aims to shape and constitute subjectivity itself. Thus the very public exercise of power through force, which aimed to terrify subjects into compliance, and of which spectacles

1 I wish to thank Bart Simon and Pascal Harvey for their helpful comments on an earlier version of this paper. A number of my arguments are further developed and supported in a forthcoming manuscript entitled *Le soupçon gothique*. See also V. de Courville Nicol (2002 a & b).

of torture were a prime example, ceded its importance to the exercise of a disciplinary power which is much more subtle, calculated and meticulous, and whose object is the soul, mind or spirit of subjects rather than their bodies (29). The ideas developed by John Locke and Cesare Beccaria can help further our understanding of this shift and its relation to Radcliffe's aesthetic of terror.

Censure, torture and impulsive forms of chastisement are condemned by Locke and Beccaria and associated with arbitrary and tyrannical forms of rule. They reject repressive types of power in favour of a type of power that shapes the values, the beliefs and consequently the behaviour of its subjects. This power is not understood as oppressive but as liberating. In fact, it is not really understood as power at all, but as moral education.

The effervescence of pedagogical thought toward the end of the eighteenth century underscores the increasing importance given to the individual internalisation of norms and values in the government of individuals and populations. The goal of moral education was to ensure subjects learned to conduct themselves in appropriate ways, and this was a sphere of particular concern in light of the spread of individualism[2] and of the growing literacy of the population (Curtis 352; Kilgour 6). While its popularisation took some time, this pedagogical ideal emerged earlier, such as in Locke's *Thoughts Concerning Education*, where the mind, understood in opposition to the body, is the object of government. Locke argues that mental pain in the form of self-discipline is the ideal substitute for physical pain in the education of children (103, 107–8, 111–13).

For Locke, education is the means through which the child internalises the external constraints that will enable him to behave in a reasonable fashion. Children's natural impulses are to

2 Important social, economic and cultural transformations during the nineteenth century produced social anxieties which were formulated in terms of a fear of individualism. The preoccupation with the moral and political isolation of egoistic individual is a counter-revolutionary theme found in the discourses of conservatives, Catholics, Saint-Simoniens, positivists, liberals and socialists alike (Lukes, *Durkheim* 196).

dominate and control others. To become an autonomous and free adult, the child must learn to sublimate (i.e., to channel in the appropriate way) these egotistical impulses by developing self-restraint and to internalise the appropriate forms of reality. In Locke's theory, it is the private self, or the spirit, rather than the body of the subject, that should constitute the object of power. Children must be coaxed rather than punished, and must learn to sublimate rather than to repress their natural impulses (cf. Kilgour 34–6 for a useful discussion of this). They must be taught, through repetition and habit-formation, that the restraint of their immediate desires will eventually bring about a greater satisfaction. This frustration of individual desire allows for the development of the social or moral adult self – a self that is in conformity with the greater needs of the social order. Should subjects fail to govern themselves in the appropriate manner, they would also fail to become free, moral and responsible citizens (Locke 109–10).

Like Locke before him, Beccaria rejected government through terror in favour of liberal government anchored in the principles of peace, security, liberty, property and equality. The Beccarian punitive economy aims at the utilitarian maximisation of collective pleasure and the minimisation of individual pain through education and the codification of offences. Crime prevention, individual liberty and social stability depend upon the individual consciousness of the consequences of an offence. In *On Crimes and Punishment*, Beccaria rejects corporal forms of punishment. He argues that liberty and independence can only be favoured if a regular and predictable legal system is developed, where individuals know the law, and where punishment is proportionate to the crime. Education should facilitate the internalisation of codified and accessible laws (88, 111, 152–53, 158).

The private self is clearly to be feared in Beccaria's model of self-government. He argues that individual passions are dangerous if they are not kept in check. Thus penalty is necessary in order to avoid the dissolution of the social bond and the return to original chaos (49). Penalties should be determined in such a way as to prevent the excess of private interests that bring about crime, without destroying the sensibility which motivates men (55). Individual freedom and social progress can only be compatible if liberty is subject to a certain amount of policing. Punishment is also to be feared. Citizens must both love and fear laws (153). This dual sensation ensures wilful compliance with rules, and fearful avoidance of crime. Beccaria argues that the idea of pain must always be in the heart of the feeble man, and should dominate the sentiment that pushes him toward crime (104). Hence, the Beccarian subject governs his desires in order to keep pain at bay. The fear of self and the fear of punishment can thus be said to be at the heart of self-government in Beccaria's felicitous society. While Beccaria condemns torture and other physical forms of violence and advocates for more 'humane' forms of punishment, in his punitive economy, pain quite simply moves inward. Fear of punishment and an ontologically suspect self act to ensure self-government.

In Locke's and Beccaria's theories, individual freedom is both a threat to and a condition of social order, harmony and progress. The 'irrational' self must be properly moulded and held in check if it is to contribute to individual and collective well-being and progress. Failure to develop a moral self will bring about decline. At the collective level, this represents a return to violence, social disorder and chaos. At the individual level, this involves a descent into madness, death or loss of liberty. Moral education is understood as the means through which subjects can develop the autonomous and adult moral selves necessary for self-government. However, the call for self-government is prompted by the fear of the consequences of non-restraint, and thus through the fear of the self as such. This forces us to question what is truly implied by courage, enlightenment and autonomy, or what the sociologist Émile Durkheim called 'the enlightened acceptance of rules' (97).

In both Lockean and Beccarian approaches to social order, self-government, or the mastery of irrational impulses, is inscribed in a dynamic of satisfaction and punishment, pleasure and pain, yet pleasure is paradoxically produced through fear. We can situate Ann Radcliffe's terror aesthetic in this context, a popular late eighteenth-century novelist whose formula for producing fear was appropriated by numerous authors in the emerging gothic tradition. In Radcliffe's aesthetic, mental pain, which is coterminous with sublime terror, is produced to bring about moral conduct and social order, and is a process through which fear is converted into pleasure. Radcliffe develops a strategy of individual government that moves through fear. Sublime terror prompts the mastery of the passions and engenders the expulsion of fear and evil excess, while ensuring moral self-government. Radcliffe's aesthetic (cf. *On the Supernatural in Poetry*) was inspired by the writings of Edmund Burke, who considered sublime terror to be a useful instrument in political and moral spheres. Terror engenders individual submission to a natural moral order and ensures individual dignity, honour and liberty.

Sublime Terror

Edmund Burke is known for his *Reflexions on the Revolution in France* (1790), which reflects his conservatism, as well as for his *A Philosophical Enquiry into the Origin of our Ideas of the Sublime and the Beautiful*, published when he was much younger. In Burke's work, the sublime[3] is no longer associated merely with

3 The use of the term *sublime* spread during the seventeenth century when the anonymous treatise *Peri Hypsous*, believed to date from the first century, was translated into English by John Hall in 1652 and in French by Nicolas Boileau in 1674 (cf. Preminger and Brogan 1231–33). The term *sublime* signifies up to *(sub)* the lintel *(limen)* (beam above a door or a window) and connotes height and greatness. Generally speaking, the sublime designates elevation, refinement and purification, as well as feelings of dignity and honour. In England, the popularisation of the expression marks the rise of subjectivism and romanticism. By the end of the eighteenth century, the sublime had become a trendy expression designating grandiose sentiments such as admiration, enthusiasm, awe and terror.

greatness and awe, but with terror. His treatise on the romantic aesthetic had a remarkable influence in England, France and Germany, and his psychological perspective of the aesthetic problem was influenced by John Locke. In his work on sublimity, Burke argues that the minute examination of the passions will enable us to understand their effects:

> I imagined that it could only be from a diligent examination of our passions in our own breasts; from a careful survey of the properties of things which we find by experience to influence those passions; and from a sober and attentive investigation of the laws of nature, by which those properties are capable of affecting the body, and thus of exciting our passions. (1)

The importance of Burke's enquiry is that it represents an attempt to understand the utility of terror in its relation to power. His theory inspired Radcliffe's gothic literary approach, whereby circumstances engendering precise and predictable passions in the reader are produced in order to elevate sensibility and purify judgment. Sublime terror is the principal emotion at the heart of this transformation. A brief incursion into some of the main ideas put forth by Burke in his enquiry will allow us to gain a better understanding of the productivity of pain in Radcliffe's gothic novel *The Mysteries of Udolpho*.

Burke makes an important distinction between positive emotions such as pleasure and pain, and emotions that constitute an attenuating distance toward pleasure and pain. For Burke, pleasure and pain are positive and separate emotions. Pleasure does not depend upon the negation of pain, any more than pain depends on the negation of pleasure:

> It must be observed that the cessation of pleasure affects the mind in three ways. If it simply ceases, after having continued a proper time, the effect is indifference; if it be abruptly broken off, there ensures an uneasy sense called disappointment; if the object be so totally lost that there is no chance of enjoying it again, a passion arises in the mind, which is called grief. [...] in grief, the pleasure is still uppermost; and the affliction we suffer has no resemblance to absolute pain, which is always odious, and which we endeavour to shake off as soon as possible. (37)

Pain and terror can be differentiated to the extent that pain acts on the mind by way of the body, whereas terror acts on the body by way of the mind. The impression of danger or threat is thus one which is distinct from that of pain for Burke, and it is through the former that the submission of individuals to the moral order must pass. This submission is a condition of moral strength, justice and wisdom. Both pain and terror can produce a sensation of delight (negative pleasure) if the first does not give way to violence and if the second does not have personal destruction as a consequence. The passions which bring about delight (the elimination of danger or of pain, or in other words relief) are sublime and are the strongest ones because they have to do with self-preservation:

> To draw the whole of what has been said into a few distinct points. The passions which belong to self-preservation, turn on pain and danger; they are simply painful when their causes immediately affect us; they are delightful when we have an idea of pain and danger, without being actually in such circumstances; this delight I have not called pleasure, because it turns on pain, and because it is different enough from any idea of positive pleasure. Whatever excites this delight, I call *sublime*. (51)

Thus, ideas of pain and danger constitute the source of the sublime for Burke:

> Whatever is fitted in any sort to excite the ideas of pain, and danger, that is to say, whatever is in any sort terrible, or is conversant about terrible objects, or operates in a manner analogous to terror, is a source of the sublime, that is, it is productive of the strongest emotion which the mind is capable of feeling. (39)

The sublime has as its sources objects that inspire uncertainty and confusion. Vacuity, darkness, solitude and silence are sublime privations. Sublime terror acts on the mind, depriving it of its capacity to act and reason:

> No passion so effectually robs the mind of all its power of acting and reasoning as fear. For fear being apprehension of pain or death, it operates in a manner that resembles actual pain. Whatever therefore is terrible, with regard to sight, is sublime too, whether this cause of terror, be endured

> with greatness of dimensions or not; for it is impossible to look on any things as trifling, or contemptible, that may be dangerous. (57)

Sublime terror is a condition of government through fear:

> Those despotic governments, which are founded on the passion of men, and principally upon the passion of fear, keep their chief as much as may from the public eye. The policy has been the same in many cases of religion. Almost all the heathen temples were dark. (59)

The utility of sublime terror for Burke is that it brings about individuals' submission and consequently allows them to reach a higher moral plane. The sublime inspires wonderment and it is much more powerful than beauty, which is weak and sentimental. Similarly, in producing terror, admiration is much more powerful than love: 'Those virtues which cause admiration, and are of the sublimer kind, produce terror rather than love. Such as fortitude, justice, wisdom, and the like. Never was any man amiable by force of these qualities' (110). Love latches on to small agreeable things, whereas admiration neighbours the magnificent and grandiose at the origin of the sublime:

> There is a wide difference between admiration and love. The sublime, which is the cause of the former, always dwells on great objects, and terrible; the latter on small ones, and pleasing; we submit to what we admire, but we love what submits to us; in one case we are forced, in the other we are flattered into compliance. (113)

Of great import for our understanding of Radcliffe's gothic aesthetic, Burke argues that ignorance brings about admiration and excites our passions. Sublime privation provokes individual submission by bypassing the awareness of ordinary people:

> Uncultivated people are but ordinary observers of things, and not critical in distinguishing them; but, for that reason, they admire more, and are more affected with what they see, and therefore express themselves in a warmer and more passionate manner. If the affection be well conveyed, it will work its effect without any clear idea; often without any idea at all of the thing which has originally given rise to it. (176)

Radcliffe's Gothic Aesthetic

In 1773, Anna and John Aikin published *On the Pleasure Derived From Objects of Terror*, where they applied Burke's theories to marvellous and supernatural stories (in Clery 80–6). The authors proposed two hypotheses to explain the pleasure felt by readers of terror. They argue that the pleasure of reading these texts is not a positive one, but rather one which results from the relief procured by the resolution of the enigma. Thus this 'pleasure' is tantamount to Burke's conception of delight, which comes about through the elimination of danger or of pain. They also argue that these stories stimulate the imagination and consequently prevent the stagnation of the mind imprisoned in the banality of everyday life. Like Burke, they considered that artificial terror constituted a good remedy for those for whom age and habit had dulled the mind. Terror provokes pain through effort and the delight of cleansing an idle spirit.

In a similar vein, Ann Radcliffe categorised gothic texts based on Burke's distinction between positive and negative emotions, the latter being equated with sublime elevation. She differentiated between the positive horror (physical and explicit) of M.G. Lewis' *The Monk*, which she condemned for its paralysing, debasing and corrupting effect, and the sublime terror (mental and implicit) of her own work, which, she argued, brings about spiritual cleansing and elevation:

> Terror and horror are so far opposite, that the first expands the soul, and awakes the faculties to a high degree of life; the other contracts, freezes, and nearly annihilates them. I apprehend, that neither Shakespeare nor Milton by their fictions, nor Mr. Burke by his reasoning, anywhere looked to positive horror as a source of the sublime, though they all agree that terror is a very high one; and where lies the great difference between horror and terror, but in the uncertainty and obscurity, that accompany the first, respecting the dreaded evil? (149–50)

Radcliffe developed a formula that would inspire countless writers in the gothic tradition. Fear and morality are intertwined throughout *Udolpho*. The production of mental pain through sublime privation and the suggestion of pain and danger are ways in which Radcliffe's novel seeks to prompt moral conduct. The novel's systematic hints at 'evil' excess in multiple forms (e.g., death, torture, rape, crime and adultery) produce a sublime terror and the heroine's submission to the rules of virtuous conduct. The heroine's multiple terrifying experiences are an exercise in moral education which eventually give way to the purification and elevation of her soul. Fear of the self is another means through which the heroine's self-government is brought about and legitimated in Radcliffe's novel. The self is represented as an object which must be feared and mastered.[4] The Radcliffean self is a disorderly one which must be organised artificially through fear. The terrifying nature of the self is posed as the very condition of the need to govern oneself.

At the beginning of the novel, the death of Emily St-Aubert's mother constitutes an opportunity in moral education. Her father wishes to impress upon her that it is her duty to restrain her sorrow: 'I have endeavoured to teach you, from your earliest youth, the duty of self-command [...]. Your sorrow is useless. Do not receive this as merely a commonplace remark, but let reason *therefore* restrain sorrow' (1: 20). Importantly, it is through constant exposure to terrifying circumstances that Emily will learn to 'overcome' her love for her mother (and her lover) and develop vir-

4 The view according to which the control of individual desire is required for social order is not universal, it is culturally and historically specific (Pfister 26–9). I argue elsewhere (2002a) that the modern conception of individuals as dangerous objects to be governed emerged in the context of a liberal-democratic logic of government. This conception is conditioned by a division between the State and civil society and by the premise that individual desire is a threat which must be contained and sublimated by autonomous and rational moral selves.

tuous self-command. Her mother's death is but the first of a number of trying circumstances. Our heroine is exposed to death, destruction and corruption from the beginning to the end of the novel. The novel's production of sublime terror is an experimental and artificially produced environment which aims to transform her into a civil being, helping her develop the classic virtues of resolution, courage, justice and wisdom, or self-command through mental pain, danger and fear.

Shortly after, M. St-Aubert himself passes on, and the cautionary advice with which he leaves his daughter sets the tone for the remainder of the novel by producing a fear of excessive sensibility and the related obligation and compulsion to contain it:

> 'Above all, my dear Emily', said he, 'do not indulge in the pride of fine feeling, the romantic error of amiable minds. Those who really possess sensibility ought early to be taught that it is a dangerous quality, which is continually extracting the excess of misery or delight from every surrounding circumstance. [...] we become the victims of our feelings, unless we can in some degree command them'. (1: 81–2)

Self-government, which is here synonymous with the mastery of passionate excess, is clearly at the heart of a moral education induced by ideas of pain and danger, punishment and dangerous surplus.

The novel leaves no room to doubt the excessive sensibility of its heroine, who faints or comes close to fainting so frequently that one is predisposed to view her state as a *disorder*. Yet the play between terror and the monstrous sensibility it provokes eventually leads to the purification of her overactive imagination. Despite her constant exposure to death threats, illicit desire and corrupt role models, her virtuous respect for convention ultimately secures the emergence of a proper understanding and freedom from terror.

Danger, superstition, falsity, degradation and oppression are the consequence of excessive sensibility, while safety, truth, dignity and liberty arise from self-command. The heroine learns that it is the danger within, rather than the danger without, that is the cause of her pain and fear. Thus when Emily sees her lover Valancourt, with whom her aunt had prohibited any meeting, she becomes aware of her own desire through his own, a warning sign she heeds by quitting his presence: 'His countenance was the mirror in which she saw her own emotions reflected, and it roused her to self-command' (1: 131). The painful frustration of her desire, of which the novel provides many more instances, ensures the safeguarding of Emily's virtue and the greater satisfaction of her desires at the end of the novel – that is, the channelling of her desire in a socially appropriate manner through her sanctioned marriage to Valancourt. The principle of Burkean delight deployed by Radcliffe is also based on the Lockean idea that the painful frustration of desire ultimately brings about a greater satisfaction, a more important reward. Thus, behaviour informed by desire is condemned, while behaviour informed by a naturalised morality is prescribed and ultimately ensures the victory of virtue and reinstatement of moral order and truth.

In the novel, the freedom of self-government rests upon one's prior subjection to chaos, excess and unpredictability, including one's own disorderly nature. While the excessive sensibility which inhabits the heroine is at the root of her flawed understanding, victimisation, oppression and ultimately, terror, it is by being subjected to it through a process of doubling that she can ultimately rise above it – provided of course that she do so by submitting to the constraints of proper behaviour. Thus, liberty is conditioned by the sublime fear of a fundamentally passionate, excessive and dangerous human nature in need of and accepting containment. In being the very space where the threat is located (in the form of sensibility, desire, fantasy, etc.), the mind becomes the socially necessary object of a moral education.

Suspense, doubt and terror are produced through sublime privations which precede the unveiling of truth. In executing her father's last wishes, Emily must burn documents that contain the key to an enigma whose resolution would have protected her from awful moments of terror. Even when her very life is in danger, Emily chooses to observe the conventions of propriety: '(Emily) disdained to tempt the innocent girl to a conduct so mean as that of betraying the private conversation of her parents' (2: 88). Or: 'Sometimes her impatience to speak to Ludovico prompted her to send Annette to call him; but a sense of the impropriety of this at midnight restrained her' (2: 111). No matter what dangers and suffering are brought about by the frustration of her desires – even the threat of death – Emily's wilful compliance with the rules of her class and gender allow her to embrace the identity of the civil being she will eventually manage to become. In the meantime, the heroine is to learn many valuable though frightful lessons, such as the dangers involved in letting one's imagination run wild:

> It was lamentable that her excellent understanding should have yielded, even for a moment, to the reveries of superstition, or rather to those starts of imagination which deceive the senses into what can be called nothing less than momentary madness. Instances of this temporary failure of mind had more than once occurred since her return home – particularly when wandering through this lonely mansion in the evening twilight, she had been alarmed by appearances which would have been unseen in her more cheerful days. To this infirm state of her nerves may be attributed what she imagined when, her eyes glancing a second time on the armchair, which stood in an obscure part of the closet, the countenance of her dead father appeared there. (1: 105)

The dire consequences of poorly governed passions are also given voice in the personage of the nun Agnes (Dame Laurentini), whose passionate excess was the cause of her murderous impulses. The same is true of Emily's aunt, who blindly marries the monstrous Montoni, through whom she is punished dearly. In order to appropriate Madame Montoni's and Emily's fortunes, Montoni keeps them captive in the Udolpho castle. Yet the terrifying conditions of their sequestration, their isolation, ignorance and the restraint of their freedom, foreground their just and virtuous judgement. Emily's aunt comes to see her husband for the monster he is, and Emily comes to pardon the undignified complicity of her aunt. The novel teaches us that adultery, crime and madness are caused by poorly governed passions.

Radcliffe's gothic aesthetic seeks to eliminate excess through its doubling and expulsion, having as a consequence the production of a sublime terror which here again prompts and legitimates the heroine's self-government while also promoting a naturalised moral order. Knowledge privation produces ambiguity, unpredictability and fear, and causes the heroine to doubt her appreciation of reality. The excesses of Emily's imagination corrupt her judgement and prevent a proper understanding of truth: 'her imagination was inflamed, while her judgment was not enlightened, and the terrors of superstition again pervaded her mind' (1: 41). Yet she eventually learns to condemn her superstitious imagination. Seemingly supernatural events are the result of circumstances and misunderstandings – the impressions of a sickly imagination – which a deciphering of truth and a rational and necessary explanation eventually redress within a transparent and causal understanding of the universe.

In sum, the production of sublime terror legitimates the need for social order and self-restraint. It might be useful to point out here that Burke condemned Rousseau's notion of liberty for its lack of boundaries. Burke only values terror – the savage and the chaotic – to the extent that it represents an excess which prompts and legitimates individual submission to order (Botting 8). Thus in *Udolpho*, those who are not limited by external constraints fall prey to insanity, crime and violence. The fear of chaos and disorder is posed as necessary to moral existence. Virtuous, autonomous and reasonable subjects are free to govern themselves because they fear their excessive and passionate nature. In Radcliffe's text, fear and pain are at the foundation of the pleasure and freedom of self-government. Sublime terror and the frustration of desire eventually give way to delightful relief and recompense through the resolution of all enigmas, the punishment of villains, and marital bliss. Terrifying excess is ultimately rationalised in a typical Radcliffean strategy – one which allows for the naturalisation of moral principles and social hierarchies involved in the production of a bourgeois middle-class subjectivity and identity. This strategy assimilates liberty to moral restraint, and oppression to unrestrained desire in a veritable pedagogy of terror where truth is masked to allow its discovery, desire repressed to allow its liberation, and fear produced to allow its containment.

Gothic Subjectivity

Gothic subjectivity sheds light on modern forms of self-government, especially with respect to the imperative of knowing and mastering the self through fear. It is through fear of the self and fear of punishment that numerous gothic heroes and heroines are prompted to conform to the social order by sublimating their desire. Failure to do so results in perversion, loss of freedom, death and madness, and is brought about by a lack or excess of fear. I do not wish to suggest that desire or interiority are extra-social, but merely that what counts as desire is what escapes or resists containment and as such poses the threat of 'ungovernability'.

The constitution of feminine bourgeois subjectivity finds a unique expression in the gothic novel. The gothic heroine deprives herself throughout the story so that the expression of her desires is ultimately in conformity with the existing moral order. However, the recompense brought about by the painful frustration of her desires is not what motivates this restraint, as she is unaware of the final outcome of her self-restraint. Rather, it is fear of her unchecked desires, and fear of punishment occasioned by transgression, which is at the heart of the sublimation of desire. Fear prompts the internalisation of the 'appropriate forms of reality', and the concomitant development of self-government.

In Charlotte Brontë's *Jane Eyre* for instance, the gothic heroine gets her reward – a legitimate nuptial contract with Mr. Rochester – precisely because she has never succumbed to her desires in spite of multiple terrifying obstacles. In the process she becomes educated, courageous and enlightened, and thus worthy of her station. The same is true of all the gothic heroines in Radcliffe's novels, and it is also true of Maud in Sheridan Le Fanu's *Uncle Silas*, and of Mina in Bram Stoker's *Dracula*, to give but a few examples.

Conversely, lack of personal restraint, occasioned through lack or excess of fear, tends to characterise the behaviour of males, the female working class, the masses and masculine females in gothic novels. The lack of self-restraint required in the sublimation of one's impulses gives way to perversion, madness and death. Such is the fate of Manfred in *The Castle of Otranto*, of Ambrosio in *The Monk*, of Catherine Earnshaw in *Wuthering Heights*, of Dorian Gray in Oscar Wilde's gothic tale, of Lucy Westernra in *Dracula*, of Victor Frankenstein in Mary Shelley's gothic novel, of Dr. Jekyll in Robert Louis Stevenson's tale and of Dr. Moreau in H.G. Wells' *The Island of Doctor Moreau*.

For gothic subjects, the 'pleasure' of self-government depends upon the displacement of mental pain through sublimation. A painful pleasure, a Burkean delight, transforms fear into pleasure through sublimation. As such, perhaps we can understand the paradox of subjects who experience pleasure in the frustration of their desires. The desire to master oneself depends upon the prior production of a subject of fear – a subject whose desire to know and master him or herself is predicated upon a fear of the self. Thus, fortitude and perseverance – the painful frustration of desire – can lead to the 'greater satisfaction' achieved through liberal forms of integration and adaptation.

It is commonplace today to understand the effects of fear in negative, repressive terms. The discourses on fear deployed by contract theorists from the Enlightenment onwards, did much to promote this understanding. They represented fear as the negative pole of liberty, reason, autonomy, truth and civility. This conception has the effect of overshadowing the central role played by fear in liberal societies, namely through its involvement in the production of subjects who govern themselves through fear.

Works Cited

Beccaria, Cesare. *On Crimes and Punishments*. 1764. Trans. Henry Paolucci. Indianapolis: Bobbs-Merrill, 1979.

Botting, Fred. *Gothic*. London: Routledge, 1996.

Burke, Edmund. *A Philosophical Enquiry into the Origin of our Ideas of the Sublime and the Beautiful*. 1757/1759. Ed. James T. Boulton. Oxford: Basil Blackwell, 1987.

Clery, Emma. *The Rise of Supernatural Fiction, 1762–1800*. Cambridge: CUP, 1995.

Curtis, Bruce. "The Speller Expelled: Disciplining the Common Reader in Canada West." *Canadian Review of Sociology and Anthropology*, 22. 3 (1985): 346–68.

de Courville Nicol, Valérie. "La production de l'homme moderne; ou le passage de la peur à l'intérieur." *Sociologie et Sociétés*, 34. 1 (2002a): 175–97.

— "Le rêve, la peur et l'empirisme psychologique dans les écrits gothiques." *Le rêve et les lumières/The Dream and the Enlightenment*. Ed. J. Schloback. Paris: Honoré Champion, ISECS Series, International 18th Century Studies, 2002b. 243–59.

Durkheim, Émile. *L'éducation morale*, Paris: Quadrige, 1992.

Preminger, Alex and T. V. F. Brogan. *New Princeton Encyclopedia of Poetry and Poetics*. Princeton: Princeton UP, 1993. 1231–33.

Foucault, Michel. *Discipline and Punish*. New York: Vintage, 1979.

Kilgour, Maggie. *The Rise of the Gothic Novel*. New York: Routledge, 1995.

Locke, John. *Thoughts Concerning Education* 1693. Ed. John W. and Jean S. Yolton. New York: OUP, 1989.

Lukes, Steven. *Émile Durkheim: His Life and Work*. London: Penguin, 1988.

Pfister, Joel. "On Conceptualizing the Cultural History of Emotional and Psychological Life in America." *Inventing the Psychological*. Ed. Joel Pfister and Nancy Schnog. London, YUP, 1997. 17–59.

Radcliffe, Ann. *The Mysteries of Udolpho*. 1784. Ed. R. Austin Freeman. 2 vols. London: J. M. Dent & Sons Ltd, 1931.

— "On the Supernatural in Poetry." *New Monthly Magazine*, 16 (1826): 145–52.

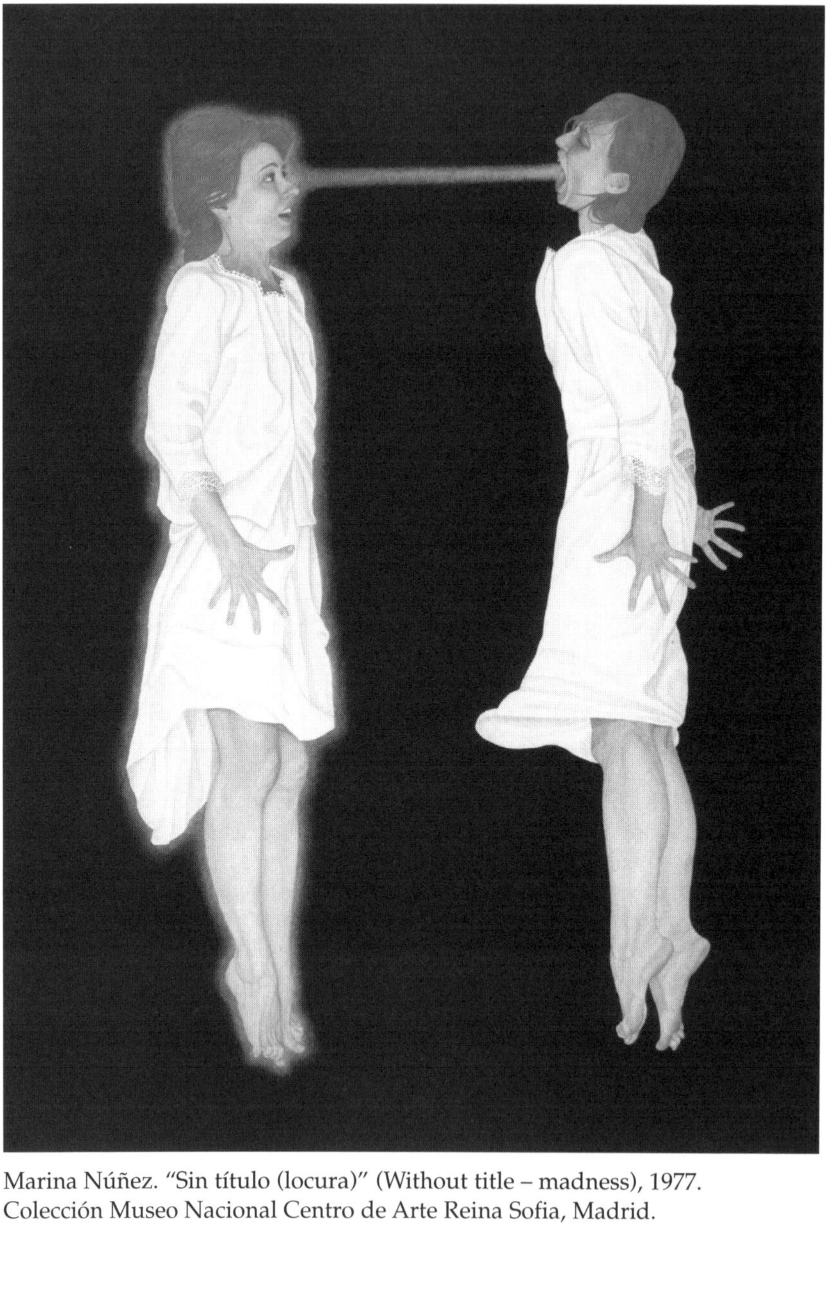

Marina Núñez. "Sin título (locura)" (Without title – madness), 1977.
Colección Museo Nacional Centro de Arte Reina Sofia, Madrid.

'To survive war, you gotta' become war.' The Productivity of Pain in Mainstream Action Films

Markus Rheindorf
University of Vienna

Preliminaries

Rather than follow what has by now become something of a custom in simply invoking Foucault's claim 'that perhaps, one day, this century will be known as Deleuzean' (165), I would like to begin by engaging with Foucault's statement, inflecting it into a specific direction by contending that perhaps, one day, mainstream cinema's action spectacles such as *Rambo: First Blood, Die Hard* or *Last Man Standing* will be known as Deleuzean. This is not to say, of course, that other films need be excluded from this claim, nor, for that matter, that they do not partake of the specific representational strategies under examination in this chapter. Westerns such as *For a Fistful of Dollars*, sport films such as the *Rocky* series and countless martial arts films in the vein of *Bloodsport* share with the above a similar reliance on the productivity of pain as a means of globally structuring the narrative. Indeed, on a different level, virtually every action film in recent film history follows the same pattern scaled down to a single, perhaps final, fight between its male protagonist and his adversary. Put briefly, this pattern, in the conventional terms of (literary) narrative analysis, could be described as an extended conflict between the (good, male) protagonist and his (evil, male) antagonist. In this conflict, evil seems to win a decisive victory over good, which, in the person of the male protagonist, is then subjected to more or less extended pain in the form of torture and/or humiliation. However, whether through sheer luck, the assistance of an outside helper, or the protagonist's own cunning, he manages to survive his torment and escapes to return – sometimes immediately, sometimes after a considerable amount of time – to finally triumph over evil.

Despite its limiting conventionality, even such an initial, classical reading already links the structural position or narrative function of pain and its productivity to questions of self and effect (or self *as* effect). To be precise, this function seems to be that pain effects a crucial change in the protagonist's identity or self, that it causes some form of change or else produces an entirely new self. Before the onset of pain, although already recognizable as the hero, he was not strong enough, not hard enough – all puns intended – to defeat evil. Only after going through excruciating pain, literally living through what is often referred to in these texts as 'hell',[1] is he able to face and overcome the challenge posed to existing structures of law and order. And we might well replace the temporal marker 'after' in the previous sentence with the explicit marker of causality it so often implies: it is only 'through' and 'because of' pain that the protagonist changes, becomes someone able to defeat the challenge. As my wording of the last sentence shows, it is deceptively easy to simply rephrase this classical analysis in Deleuzean terms, claiming that the male protagonist's identity *is* the productivity of pain insofar as it is pain which produces his subjectivity. But such a position would have accomplished little more than an appropriation of terminology, while it would remain based upon a series of Cartesian dualisms of the kind that Deleuze so violently rejects.

1 As usual, the *Rambo* films are representative in this respect: in *Rambo: First Blood II*, one character makes the point to another that '[W]hat you call hell, Rambo calls home'.

Since this false start – intentionally produced here in order to highlight the degree to which the notion of 'productivity' requires a rethinking of the subject, the body and their relation to social structure in Deleuzean terms – has never rejected the split of self into body and mind, and given the immediacy of the protagonist's recovery from pain, such a reading must assume nothing less than a victory of mind over body. Whether pain is then seen as a redemptive force, a cleansing fire that purges the body to purify the mind – leading to a phoenix-like rebirth of the male self through pain – or simply as an external force hardening and steeling the male protagonist's self to superhuman degrees is ultimately beside the point. Leaving aside for now the ideological implications of such readings, which put pain squarely and unproblematically in the service of the status quo, this position fails to make clear the operations or abstract machines through which pain is effective upon the subject, nor can it accommodate the deterritorializing effect of Deleuzean flows and intensities upon the socially structured subject. It thus fails to provide an account of the conditions under which the deterritorializing flow of pain can produce an even more structured subject, one in which all structured barriers to flows are literally hardened. In film, this 'steeling' finds its visual correlative in the hardening of the always already muscular body of the male protagonist which parallels the narrative moment outlined above (see the later sections of this chapter for a more detailed account of the significance of the body in a Deleuzean reading of the productivity of pain).

In the absence of any easy solution to the conceptual problematic outlined above, the following pages will take as their task a retracing of this intentional false start, taking a detour through both Deleuzean theory and a reading of popular action films that is implicitly deconstructive, seeking out the ruptures in these texts as much as those of the male protagonist's identity as it becomes exposed to the productivity of pain. It should perhaps be pointed out that my choice of filmic texts quite obviously privileges the popular, lowbrow entertainment products of corporate capitalism above both the independent and the avant-garde for several reasons beyond that of cultural relevance. These derive from Deleuze's (1986, 1989) own theorization of film as an enveloping event rather than a form of representation and are furthermore related to his concept of the action image (and its crisis) as well as an understanding of films as effective machines. The latter aspect, in particular, offers a venue for exploring the apparently enormous effective potential of the partly religious, partly mythological resonances of representations of pain as a purifying, elevating force effecting a rebirth of one kind or another for the male subject.

The Deleuzean subject

Once we acknowledge that in speaking of the 'productivity' of pain we are implicitly conceiving of the term in analogy to the 'productivity of desire' in Deleuze's writing, we face the task of going back farther and farther in making explicit the unspoken underpinnings of any such reading of the productivity of pain. And because Deleuze's philosophy is ultimately one of the subject, every notion in Deleuzean thought finally relates back to his understanding of subjectivity as 'permanent becoming'. Like the deconstructed subject, the Deleuzean subject is not simply socially determined, but 'in process' and productive, a 'subject-in-process', an effective determinant within the context in which it is effectively determined. Foregrounding the notion of becoming within a field of intensities rather than individual agency, Deleuze's philosophy of immanence is nevertheless profoundly affirmative in so far as it implies an ethics of becoming constantly what one is not.

Such an ethics of change and active joy seems to resonate with the general recognition that there are moments in contemporary culture, especially in popular film, that allow more fluid becomings in which categories such as gender are not a determining factor.[2] In such a Deleuzean universe, which is itself in constant flux, identities are neither fixed nor intersubjectively determined, and a fictional character's mode of being is one of permanent becoming. Indeed, identity appears to be a malleable thing in films like *Rambo: First Blood*, something that can be fashioned, albeit mostly by an always already existing and seemingly self-determining self responding to circumstances at least initially beyond its control. Thus, when John Rambo asserts that 'in order to survive war, you gotta' *become* war', he is not only acknowledging the fact that flows of intensities such as war (or what Deleuze would call a military machine) form his identity, but is also phrasing his convictions in terms strikingly similar to Deleuze's theory of the subject. And yet, mainstream action films such as *Rambo: First Blood* and popular culture in general cannot be comfortably considered to be entirely Deleuzean as they in many ways reaffirm traditional molar structures such as that of the private and self-determining subject.[3]

It is in any case important to realize that the subject as the private subject, even if socially determined, is no longer a category in Deleuze's writing. Especially in the method of schizoanalysis (Deleuze & Guattari 1985), the subject is not individual, not discursive and not ideological. It is produced before the significations of ideology at the level of the breaks and flows of material desire, not merely in process, but nomadic and polyvocal. The Deleuzean subject thus provides a measure and consummation of that which produces it as a residue. But the state of fluc-

2 For a number of essays dedicated to determining just how Deleuzean the twentieth century and, in particular, its popular culture, is, see the special issue of *Theory, Culture and Society* edited by Mike Featherstone.

3 See also Rosi Braidotti's (1997) essay on 'Meta(l)morphoses: The Becoming Machine', in which she argues that Deleuze's scheme does not correspond to the reality of mainstream film or *vice versa*.

tuation of the subject is by no means an exception in Deleuzean thought. In rhizomatics, Deleuze & Guattari's strategy of cultural analysis in *Anti-Oedipus* and *A Thousand Plateaus*, a similar vocabulary of flows, lines of flight and intensities is used in a process of drawing lines of connections, links between points within a multidimensional and multidirectional field in order to map out reality in terms of the productive relations between points. While poststructuralism can be said to exclude the other from its discourse, rhizomatics is thus entirely a philosophy of the other. As anything is defined by the connections it has with other points, by its field of effects, there are only others, only the real.[4]

Within this larger theoretical framework, it becomes possible to explore a notion of identity without selfhood, of subjectivity as a nomadic and schizophrenic becoming. There are two main aspects to becoming in Deleuze's writing which ultimately allow one to theorize the connection between identity and pain, both of which are constitutive of identity. The first of these is Deleuze and Guattari's conception of desire as pure productivity, which can offer a line of flight away from humanist notions of identity and selfhood while simultaneously challenging psychoanalysis' heritage of Cartesian dualisms. The second concept of importance in this regard is the somewhat elusive notion of the 'body without organs', which further destabilizes the centrality of the self and the other – or else subject and object in Freudian theories of sexuality – in their interdependence.

4 For the somewhat problematic relation of the Deleuzean subject in society to cultural studies and its tradition of Western Marxism, see Grossberg (*Bringing* 90). In his attempted mediation between the two, Grossberg equates productivity with effects or, more accurately, 'effectivities', and concludes that Deleuze's conception might be used productively in cultural studies. On a similar note, Braidotti also sees the concept of becoming and of the deterritorializing forces of desire that can open up the classical notion of the subject as very useful for cultural studies and the analysis of all kinds of new subjectivities in cultural texts.

Keeping in mind Deleuze's ethos of 'permanent becoming-revolutionary', to which I shall return in greater detail at a later point, it thus becomes possible to connect the ideas of politics and hypercapitalism developed by Kenneth Surin to film and the cinema. The question, then, is whether there can be any machinic points within the hypercapitalist film (and media) industry that could contribute to a 'permanent becoming-revolutionary' of the image and sound. While Surin's argument remains rather abstract in itself and since, as Millet argues, for Deleuze 'philosophy should have a horror of abstraction' (53), I will take the issues raised by Surin as a cue to look at concrete films (or media events) as singular multiplicities in order to determine what kinds of becoming take place in mainstream action films. The detour I take in order to do so therefore continues with conceiving of pain as a deterritorializing flow similar to – and as an agent of – Deleuzean desire.

Deleuzean desire and pain

Deleuze's conception of desire as pure productivity implies and is initially based upon a critique of the history of desire in philosophical thought which he sees as inextricably linked to Descartes' cogito and a series of Cartesian dualisms (soul-body, thought-extension, statement-enunciation). Dualism, for Deleuze, is radically inimical to thought, as it denies the essence of thought as a process. The source of any such dualism is the flattening of all statements of thought by what Deleuze calls 'a speculative, Oedipal apparatus' ('Dualism' 95). It is this apparatus which needs to be recognized in the Cartesian cogito, which claims that every statement is the production of a subject. Implied by this first aspect is a second point: that every statement splits the subject that produces it into a subject of the statement and the subject of enunciation (in this, Deleuze regards Lacan as 'the last Cartesian'). This proposition follows directly from the first, because if it is true that a statement is produced by a subject, then for that very reason this subject will be divided into the subject of enunciation and the subject of the statement. This is what the literal process of the cogito consists of, and while it is possible to say 'I think, therefore I am,' one cannot say 'I walk, therefore I am.' This amounts to the first and, to Deleuze, most insidious dualism, that of mind and body. However, in the century that Foucault saw as Deleuzean, Deleuze himself is obviously not the only one to be disputing the sovereignty of the cogito. At least on a surface level, the cinema of the action film is a cinema of bodies in action, of bodies that walk, fight or operate a machine gun. John Rambo, Rocky Balboa and John McClane, to name but a few of the better known examples, all act or fight with their bodies, therefore they are.

In a classical reading, however, the emergence of a stronger identity in mainstream action films can be understood only as the result of pain working within and upon the mind/body dualism of the Cartesian cogito. In this view, pain is seen as structurally and directly related to the victory of mind over body in the case of the male protagonist, a defeat of the crude matter of the body which brings about a stronger, more masculine self. Framed within a mind/body dialectic, mind can only manifest itself as body in action films and is thus at first indistinguishable from it. Only when pain begins to work upon the body does the mind (made manifest as body) triumph over the body because it is filled with, made to be equivalent with pain and thus 'cleansed' or 'purified', leaving behind only the mind (as body) freed of the body.

Not only would such a reading fall prey to dualism's equation of identity, subjectivity and ultimately also of human agency with the mind and thus split it entirely from the body, but would also be incapable of theorizing the relation of these multiple bodies to each other: the body without pain, the body in pain, and the body that remains the site of agency even after the mind has been supposedly freed from it. Pain would thus be seen as effectively splitting the mind and thus the 'I' from the body, an operation in which it parallels that of the cogito and, by extension, that of desire in Cartesian thought. As has already been suggested, Deleuze links the cogito to the history of the concept of desire not only because of their similar conception, but because thinking and desiring are ultimately the same thing to him. More specifically, Deleuze sees a vicious circle of maledictions informing the history of desire in philosophical thought, especially in what he calls 'this rotten theory of desire, word for word' of psychoanalysis ('Dualism' 98). Desire is thus completely ensnared, taken up in a circle which Deleuze reconstructs following Plato's method in the *Phaedo*. This circle is characterized by a tendency of linking desire to a beyond, whether it's that of lack, pleasure or 'jouissance', and of posing the dualism between the subject of enunciation and the subject of the statement.[5]

The first malediction in this – and the first arc in the circle 'damning' desire – equates desire with lack; and once desire is linked to lack, so Deleuze, one is immediately in the domain of dualisms, has in fact already accepted the basis of all dualism and 'non-thought' (95). While this first arc links directly to the cogito, there are more underhanded ways of reintroducing lack into desire, either through the Other, or through the dualism implied by pleasure. Deleuze rejects the relation between desire and pleasure as 'a completely rotten conception', recognizing in this the second malediction of desire (95). This second arc derives from the assumption that desire is fundamentally aimed at an Other, open to a transcendence, and can supposedly be fulfilled. However, what can fulfill it will never be truly that toward which it tends, except in appearance, but the Other, forever unattainable and transcendental. What is said to come to fulfill or satisfy it and

5 According to Deleuze, the relation between the split of the subject (of enunciation and of the statement) and desire is forged at the level of the Cartesian cogito, which also constructs a circle in the form of a system of statements in which the 'I' is the subject of the statement ('Dualism' 102).

which gives it a pseudo-immanence is what is called a state of pleasure and is to Deleuze only a different way of 'cursing and liquidating desire' (96). In this second arc, however, it is already understood that this immanence is a false immanence, since desire has been fundamentally defined in relation to a transcendence, and this fulfillment is, *à la lettre*, an illusion. Thus, in this second malediction of desire, pleasure is introduced as a matter of calming desire for a moment, of having provisionally 'done with desire' before it begins again (101).[6]

While pleasure, in its conception as a discharge, obliterates desire for a while, the third malediction – and the arc which closes the circle – links desire with the impossible transcendence of the Other. As desire remains irreducible to states of pleasure, even if one introduces these states of rest or satisfaction, which can only satisfy desire in appearance, it must be reaffirmed in the mode of transcendence as the impossible jouissance-death relation. In this last arc of the vicious circle, pleasure is ultimately not the satisfaction of desire, but its opposite: an exasperation of the process that derives desire of its own immanence, i.e., its own productivity. Deleuzean desire, on the other hand, simultaneously loses any link with lack, pleasure and jouissance. It is conceived as the production of a flow, defining its own irreducible field of immanence and as such is effectively constitutive of the multiplicities that populate it. It is a multiplicity in which, significantly, any splitting of the subject into a subject of enunciation and a subject of the statement becomes strictly impossible.

As an alternative to Lacan's dystopian version of the deluded and hapless oedipal subject, the Deleuzean subject thus implies a utopian politics of polyvalent desire no longer conceived as re-

6 Deleuze's rejection of the idea of pleasure is ultimately based on his reading of Freud and his conception of desire as a disagreeable tension requiring a discharge. Discarding the notion of pleasure is, in fact, pivotal to Deleuze's aim of recasting desire as a positive force productive in its own right.

ducible to the sexual or the libidinal, in which 'mal-adjustments' such as masochism or schizophrenia are seen not as pathology but as subversive disorderings of bourgeois thought processes. Such disorderings are effected through a disruption or restructuring of Deleuze's 'desir-ing machines' modeled after Melanie Klein's part-objects and Freudian/Lacanian partial drives. In fact, the 'machine' occupies an important place in the Deleuzean conception of desire as it is through such machines that desire operates on the Oedipally unorganized 'body without organs', structuring it into the 'socius'. In contrast to Freudian or Lacanian desire, Deleuzean desire thus invests objects directly, rather than becoming enmeshed in forms of ideology and representation.

The same argument could be made for pain, insofar as it too operates upon the subject as a machine without the pre-mediation of representation or ideology. Nevertheless, the notion of a 'subject in pain' presents a number of conceptual difficulties which I can only begin to work through at this point. To begin with, it would appear that pain, unlike Deleuzean desire, is an intensity that works directly upon the body from without, while Deleuzean desire seems to emanate from within the subject (a misconception addressed below). In this traditional view, pain would thus be seen at best as a state, a process or quality where the subject can be immersed in (and must at some point emerge from). But this division into an interior and an exterior is based upon the underlying dualism of the cogito criticized and rejected by Deleuze as the split of the subject into the subject of enunciation and the subject of the statement. Deleuzean desire does, in fact, not originate in the subject, even though it flows through and from the body without organs. In this respect, pain does not differ from it as a productivity, as both are deterritorializing forces projected into the subject. Like the desir-ing subject, the suffering or pain-ing subject is the site of a productivity or an intensity manifesting itself in the body without organs. If we are to conceive of pain as a flow or intensity much like desire, it must also hold that pain is not reducible to lack, not even a lack of power (i.e., the power to avert pain). If, indeed, we were to reduce it to the Nietzschean will to power (or Deleuzean desire), this would miss the quality of pain as a distinct productivity. Pain, much like desire, is not the absence of pleasure, but a presence, an intensity constituting its own field of effects.

As an intensity or productivity in the Deleuzean sense, pain can furthermore mark a machinic point of a group or a given collectivity. Such a point would indicate, within a group and at a given moment, the maximum of deterritorialization as well as, and at the same time, its power of innovation. Significantly, this machinic point of deterritorialization (manifesting itself in the pain-ing subject) is reterritorialized in qualified machines, in this or that military machine in its discursive representation, and then, in the discursive machine of mainstream action film becomes productive of new statements that are affirmative of social structure (or, rather, of the *socius* as the body structured within society).

In Deleuze and Guattari's conception of the relationship between desire and the social system (which they formulate as a critique of Wilhelm Reich's materialist psychiatry), the interdependence of the two consists of more than the deterritorializing effect that desire can have upon social structures, Oedipal or otherwise. In fact, it is the Oedipal stage that first codes and reduces the multiplicity of desiring-machines into a subject that is based on socially exploitable genital sexuality and that mirrors the authoritarian form of the State. However, the decoding tendency of the capitalist system constantly opens up new markets of desire which it must then rigidly control in order to survive. Based on Deleuze and Guattari's ethics for a postmodern, deconstructed society, the practice of schizoanalysis in fact consists of pushing the capitalist process further, removing the limits capitalism places on these operations of decoding or deterritorialization in order to free the desiring machines and dismantle the subject as mirror of the State: 'At capitalism's limit the deterritorialized *socius* gives way to the body without organs, and the decoded flows throw themselves into desiring-production' (Deleuze & Guattari,

Anti-Oedipus 140).[7] In this sense, then, desire can become revolutionary or utopian insofar as it can be involved in the delegitimating of a ruling group. As has already been indicated, pain has a similarly deterritorializing effect on the organ-ized body and therefore lends itself to a similar reading as utopian in the sense that it functions not as a group fantasy, but as an agent of the real productivity of desire, making it possible to disinvest the current social field, to de-institutionalize it (Pisters, 'Possibilities'). We must, however, ask ourselves under which conditions and as part of which machines pain can become productive of such deterritorialization – and why, in mainstream action films, it seems to have the reverse effect. These questions, I believe, inevitably lead to the body without organs (and its correlate, the *socius*) as well as to a theorization of the relation between the body without organs and the flow of pain.

The body without organs and the deterritorializing productivity of pain

> It's a question of life and death [...] sadness and joy. It is where everything is played out.
>
> (Deleuze & Guattari, *Thousand* 151)

First appearing in Deleuze's *The Logic of Sense* and then modified in the two volumes of *Capitalism and Schizophrenia*, co-authored with Felix Guattari, the notion of the body without organs is crucially tied to 'becoming revolutionary' by means of deterritoriali-

7 Deleuze and Guattari's *A Thousand Plateaus* takes the completion of this decoding operation (deterritorialization, the scrambling of all codes, which subsumes the deconstruction of metaphysics that Derrida undertakes) as its starting point, and proceeds to create concepts for a world free of hierarchy and dialectical opposition.

zation. The body without organs is a body which 'is not at all a notion or a concept but a practice, a set of practices' (Deleuze & Guattari, *Thousand* 149); rather than a pre-existing entity, it is something that can only be 'made' by the subject.[8] In fact, Deleuze and Guattari make the point that there is no single body without organs, there are as many as you like. As a thing to produce or fabricate, the body without organs does not come ready-made and cannot exist until you try to produce it: 'As long as you have not made your body without organs, alone, with someone else, with *n* people, nothing is possible, you have to find your own' (149).

Regarding the relation between the subject and the body without organs, Deleuze and Guattari argue that subjectivity needs to be seen as something grafted onto the disconnected sites of desire rather than as the source of desire. While desire does appear to emanate from the body without organs – as, for instance, when Deleuze and Guattari describe it as 'the field of immanence of desire, the plane of consistency specific to desire' (154) – the body without organs is fully realized only when these desiring machines break down. The body without organs is thus that which resists the organization of the body that implies an individualized subject to which all these organs are a 'part of', as opposed to being autonomous producers of desire. It is consequently not a body stripped of organs, but a body upon which that what serves as organs (or machines) is distributed; it is therefore 'opposed less to organs as such than to the organization of the organs insofar as it composes an organism' (30).

As a potentially revolutionary practice, the body without organs thus functions as a projective site for the workings of the organs or desiring-machines whose socially productive nature is

8 Rather than the more negative view of the body without organs in *Anti-Oedipus* as a non-productive entity that interrupts flows and arrests desire, I draw mostly on the later *A Thousand Plateaus*, in which it is depicted as a potentially revolutionary force productive in its own right.

always imposed upon the unstructured body without organs. It is therefore also that which is itself non-productive but into which desiring production sends its lines of flight. As the surface of inscription for every statement or for every desire, it 'is made in such a way that it can be occupied, populated only by intensities' (153). And while intensities pass and circulate in it, it is 'not a scene, a place, or even a support upon which something comes to pass' (153). Rather, as 'it produces and distributes them in a *spatium* that is itself intensive, lacking extension' (153), the body without organs can be said to cause intensities to pass. Therefore it is not space, nor is it in space: 'it is matter that occupies space to a given degree – to the degree corresponding to the intensities produced. It is non-stratified, unformed, intense matter, the matrix of intensity' (153). When Deleuze and Guattari furthermore claim that '[T]he BwO is what remains when you take everything away', what they are thinking of in particular is 'precisely the phantasy, and significances and subjectifications as a whole' into which the process of psychoanalysis translates everything, converting it into structure: '[I]t royally botches the real, because it botches the BwO' (151). In this sense, constructing a body without organs does not simply go beyond psychoanalysis, but reverses its operation (150).

While there is no such thing as a manual or even a guideline for constructing a body without organs, Deleuze and Guattari touch upon several examples of successfully constructed bodies without organs. And although Antonin Artaud's suicide may be the most prominent of these instances, most of them are far more careful experiments conducted in the field of literature. Thus they say of Kafka or Castaneda that they, too, construct a body without organs, inventing for themselves a deterritorializing machine in the form of their writing. Regardless of the specific means (which will each yield a specific body without organs, as there are as many different ones as there are ways of constructing one), strategies for making a body without organs require for it to be freely traversed by the lines of desiring production and be populated by intensities. In this, the desert serves Deleuze and Guattari as a model for a surface used in the production of statements, but only on the condition that certain things take place on it. Constructing a body without organs thus becomes a matter of 'populating the desert', of being populated with intensities such as desire, pain or perhaps war. It is not to play at being what one is not, but to be populated with it. Since to play is not enough, one has to pass through other experimentations, to undertake the process of undoing the organization of the body in favor of something else, an (at least partially) unorganized body that does not (fully) integrate with existing social structures.

At first glance, it would appear that such a body without organs does not, cannot exist in mainstream action films, which are characteristically filled with well structured and organized bodies such as those of police officers or soldiers. Even if there is a mal-adjustment, as in *Rambo: First Blood*, this mismatch between the body of the male protagonist and social structure is not caused by the absence of structure, but by their inadequacy to present circumstances. Rambo has 'become war' in order to survive war, he has populated with the intensities of war and made it the site of a military machine and a war machine.

The first *Rambo* film actually complicates the usual pattern, partly because it is based on a novel and is set not in times of war but 'back home' after the war is already over. The film's action sets in some time after John Rambo has returned from Vietnam, where, after he had 'become war', his identity was meaningful within the social structures of the army. 'Back there', he explains this fit between *socius* and social structure, 'I could fly a gunship, I could drive a tank, I was in charge of million dollar equipment'. The mismatch is between the structures he has maintained grafted onto his body without organs and civilian life: 'For me civilian life is nothing! In the field we had a code of honor, you watch my back, I watch yours. Back here there's nothing'. The actual mismatch, however, is poignantly illustrated through the fact that Rambo, the perfect 'killing-machine', 'can't even hold a job washin' cars'. His re-action to this mis-fit is not simply violent – in Japanese, 'rambo' actually means 'violence' – it effectively re-creates the social structures of war – a war machine – in order to re-establish a match between John Rambo's *socius* and his surroundings. This manifests itself, for instance, when Rambo desperately reassures himself that there are, in fact, 'no friendly civilians' out there, and in an extended monologue in which he insistently denies that the social structures around him have, in fact, changed:

> Nothing is over!!! Nothing!!! You just don't turn it off! […]. And I come back to the world and I see all those maggots at the airport, protesting me, spitting. Calling me baby killer and all kinds of crap! Who are they to protest me?! Who are they?! Unless they've *been me* and been there and know what the hell they're yelling about!

But the film depicts more than simply the psychotic denial of a Vietnam veteran; it shows how the structures that regulate the flow of intensities within the subject can actually force social structures to change, to adapt to John Rambo's initially mal-adjusted *socius*. Only then is he 'captured' and humiliated (in this case by a small town's over-zealous sheriff), in other words: exposed to the productivity of pain. In effect, the same process is re-iterated in both sequels to the first *Rambo* film, with the exception that corresponding social structures are now found in some geographical and political other: first Vietnam in *Rambo: First Blood II*, and then Afghanistan in *Rambo III*. In the first of these sequels, Rambo's superior officer Trautman tells him 'to try and forget the war […] the old Vietnam's dead'.[9] Since 'the old Vietnam' as a concept is, of course, what John Rambo has 'become', his defiant but quite logical reply is that 'I'm alive, it's still

9 According to the novel's author David Morrell, Samuel Trautman, the man who claims to have 'made' Rambo, was named after Uncle Sam, implying that it was the United States government that created the soldier John Rambo.

alive'. In all three films, as in most mainstream action films, the male protagonist is submitted to pain *in extremis* before the structures of his identity become hard enough for him to withstand and overcome his enemies. John McClane in *Die Hard* is also subjected to torture-like pain when he has to run bare-footed across a floor covered in broken glass – only then, at the limit of the deterritorialized *socius*, does the man who formulated his aim in life as 'never to have to say I'm sorry' tell his wife that he is, in fact, sorry. This point marks the onset of a body without organs, the dis-organization of his well-structured masculine identity that precedes his reversion to a structured body of super-human hardness. Tellingly, his adversary Hans Gruber puts McClane's identity in direct relation to the popular image of the American male created by mainstream action films in the following lines: 'But you have me at a loss. You know my name but who are you? Just another American who saw too many movies as a child? Another orphan of a bankrupt culture who thinks he's John Wayne? Rambo? Marshall Dillon?'

As has already been suggested, Deleuze and Guattari recognize in masochism and its application of pain a viable strategy of deterritorialization, and thus see 'the masochist [as] us[ing] suffering [or pain] as a way of constituting a body without organs and bringing forth a plane of consistency of desire' (155). And while they concede that 'there are other ways, other procedures than masochism, and certainly better ones', this 'is beside the point [...] it is enough that some find this procedure suitable for them' (155). Deleuze and Guattari's choice of the more general term 'suffering' instead of the more specifically physical intensity of 'pain' is also of importance here as it indicates that mental suffering (or pain) can be productive in more or less the same way as physical pain. Indeed, humiliation and other forms of mental suffering and pain are also present alongside physical pain in most mainstream action films, including those discussed here. In all these cases, a certain distribution of intensities of pain is being drawn on the body of the male protagonist, lines of deterritorialization following deterritorialized intensities, dissolving the male body's structures or organ-ization as the *socius*. In the process of undoing the organization of the social body, the protagonist thus approaches or approximates the construction of a body without organs as described by Deleuze and Guattari. And in all this, the subject becomes, *à la lettre*, a nomadic flow which itself traverses the lines of deterritorialization, the intensities of pain and desire.

Now it is one thing to maintain that the deterritorialized and deterritorializing intensities of pain crisscrossing the body to the point at which it becomes a body without organs have to be seen as a subversive and therefore positive force within a Deleuzean framework. It is quite another to claim the same role for the represented productivity of pain within a mainstream action film which, to say the least, tends to react rather inimically to any threat to the established molar structures of society.[10] In such an analysis, we need to return to the notion of pain as a machinic point; as Deleuze and Guattari put it, the significance of knowing a machinic point lies in the fact that it marks the maximum of deterritorialization on a given body. The male protagonists in mainstream action films recede violently from this point of maximum deterritorialization and, in reverting to an organized body, in fact overcompensate for the temporary loss of structure by producing even stronger structures. The reason for this reversion is not primarily ideological, which is to say it is not ideological in cause, though it may be in its effects. It takes place in the body without organs and is thus effective, preceding ideology. On a cautionary note, Deleuze and Guattari write that 'overdose is a danger' in the experimentation of deterritorializing of one's body:

10 A considerable number of analyses, conducted in various veins of method and theory, of which Elsaesser and Buckland's deconstructive reading of *Die Hard* can perhaps be taken as exemplary, have offered rich and detailed accounts of precisely this ideological work of mainstream action films and their effectivity within specific historical contexts.

'You don't do it with a sledgehammer, you use a very fine file' (160). What you would do, then, is to 'invent self-destructions that have nothing to do with the death-drive. Dismantling the organism never meant killing yourself, but rather opening the body to connections [...]' (160). Thus, what seems at first glance paradoxical as an effect of the deterritorializing productivity of pain is really the consequence of its misapplication. As Deleuze and Guattari put it, '[Y]ou don't reach the BwO [...] by wildly destratifying [...]. If you free it with too violent an action, if you blow apart the strata without taking precautions, then [...] you will be killed, plunged into a black hole, or even dragged toward catastrophe' (160). What is more, they have a very accurate idea of what happens 'if you throw the strata into demented or suicidal collapse': it is 'the worst that can happen' because it 'bring[s] them back down on us heavier then ever' (161); which is to say, it causes the subject to revert to socially productive structures and actually overcompensate for the temporary threat of the loss of structure by making these structures 'heavier than ever'.

Produced by machines

If it is true that filmic texts are, in Deleuzean terms, 'statements' and that there are no individual statements (although there are singular multiplicities), as no statement can be produced by the singular, it follows that statements concerning the productivity of pain (or, specifically, the relation between pain and social structure as it exists in the form of the *socius*) are equally produced by machinic assemblages, or what amounts to the same thing, 'collective agents of enunciation' (Deleuze, 'Dualism' 105). This is of course true only on the condition that we understand that 'collective' does not mean 'peoples', but that Deleuze's collective agents are all multiplicities, whatever their nature.

Bearing the above in mind, it needs to be pointed out that there are numerous other aspects to the issue of pain in mainstream action films which have so far been neglected. Among them are issues of the social productivity of film as well as of the cinema as specific machinic assemblages that are effective rather than representational. If I have concentrated so far on making visible the becomings within the diegesis and the intensities projected within representational machines rather than the machinic assemblages within which they operate, this is because they are related to an extraordinary extent to a Deleuzean conception of becoming and productivity. And yet, the representational machines alluded to above have the property of creating the illusion of fixing the subject; at the same time as depicting a subject's becoming, they also confirm its submission to the cogito and turn it into an organism, the *socius* or organized body within society.

On a broader societal level, the task of describing the productivity of pain in mainstream action films would thus be no less than accounting for the way these films as specific machinic agents of enunciation effectively produce variable statements in the specific circumstances of the late twentieth century; of describing how these statements are necessarily desires (to prevent deterritorialization) on an entirely different, extra-diegetic and non-representational level; and of delineating, as I have done, how, within this production of statements, the illusion of a subject is engendered as split into a subject of enunciation and a subject of the statement.

Cinema, the movement image and the spectator

It is precisely to the role and productivity of action films as effective machines in turn producing effects on the body of the spectator that I want to focus on in the remainder of this chapter. At least initially, theorizing action films as effective machines should be seen as a way of acknowledging (if not exhaustively explaining) the popularity of these films as such, as well as of their articulations of a particular kind of male identity produced by pain *in extremis*. We can thus begin by saying that effect is produced when the machinic point of deterritorialization (brought about by pain) is re-territorialized in this or that representative machine, or in this or that effective machine, thus becoming productive of new statements. As Deleuze and Guattari (1987) have pointed out, there are always necessarily culturally and ideologically interpretable systems of indices under which re-territorializations are made in such qualified machines. Needless to say, these systems of indices are highly contextual and therefore require a more detailed examination of the cultural and historical contexts of each singular multiplicity than is reasonably possible here; what is possible, however, is to point, again, to the many ideological analyses of mainstream action films, such as Elsaesser and Buckland (2002) on *Die Hard* and Storey (2003) on *Rambo: First Blood* and a number of other 'Vietnam movies' of the 1980s, for an approximation of these indices.

And while the notion of effect (as worked out, for instance, in Grossberg) rather than ideology or representation seems best suited to the task of grasping the workings of machines such as the cinema, such a framework of analysis can only be applied if brought within a Deleuzean perspective of the cinema itself. Deleuze has, of course, already attempted this task in the form of his two volumes on cinema that can be said to constitute his theory of film (or a philosophy of film more generally).[11] What

11 In the words of Elsaesser and Buckland, we might say that the Deleuze of the two cinema books discards the categories of conventional film analysis and disregards the niceties of reasoned argument so violently 'that one either learns how to float on his prose or soon drowns in it' (270). Also relevant besides the two cinema books are those co-authored with Felix Guattari, as numerous concepts developed in these works have also been applied to the cinema (cf. Pisters, *Micropolitics* and Buchanan).

remains to be done at this point is to establish a link between what has been said above concerning the articulation of the productivity of pain in mainstream action films, Deleuze's notion of the movement image and a particular moment in contemporary film known as the crisis of the action image.

As might be expected, Deleuze submits traditional film theory to a radical critique for conceiving of film (or the cinema) as static, photographic images that move, to which he opposes the notions of movement-images and time-images. These are for Deleuze not bound to a specific material support, but realities in their own right, part of the energies, the flux and intensities and effectivities that make up Deleuze's sheets of time. That is partly why, to Deleuze, the cinema experience is an enveloping reality, at once actual and virtual, mental and somatic, made up of what he calls 'optical sound situations' rather then merely or even predominately visual perceptions. The cinema – rather than the film as text – is thus seen as a succession of open events involving the spectator, rather than as coded representations of a reality that does not participate in the actual viewing/screening experience.

Deleuze's theory of the cinema effectively counters the linguistic-semiotic trend in film theory, which reduces cinema to the filmic and thus to the textual, by recasting film in a language of sensory immediacy and bodily perception. In the process of doing so, he deploys Peirce's theory of signs against Metzian filmolinguistics and against the Lacanian system which makes cinematic desire orbit around the 'lack' rooted in the gap between an imaginary signifier and its signified. In furthermore drawing on Bergson as a philosopher of becoming, for whom being and matter are never stable, Deleuze conceives of matter and movement as imbued with and inseparable from consciousness as itself material. What interests him are therefore not images of something which would constitute a diegesis, but rather the images themselves, caught up in the flux of time, which returns us to his understanding of film as event rather than representation. The cinema to Deleuze is more than either art or representation (rejecting the dualism of traditional film theory, usually termed 'formalism' and 'realism'). Instead, it is to him a philosophical instrument *per se*, a generator of concepts and a producer of texts which renders thought in audiovisual terms, not in language but in 'blocks of movement and duration'. Deleuze's theory of cinema is therefore not so much about cinema as a medium but about the concepts that the cinema itself triggers and the ways in which it gives rise to new connections between fields and disciplines. It is thus as much a matter of cinematizing philosophy as of theorizing the cinema.

Since Deleuze simultaneously moves from the spectator as self to the body as a site of intensities, providing the fields of negotiating effectivities in the cinema experience, the concept of the body without organs also comes to redefine the issue of 'identification' within the cinema as an effective machine. The body becomes not only a topographical 'site' for an inscription of the cinema and its different kinds of textuality, but also emerges as the locus of energies and intensities emanating from it and oscillating between spectator and screen. In the cinema event, the body is thus both foundational and constructed, a given and the result of the image. As a consequence, it would be possible, at least theoretically, to construct for oneself a body without organs by means of the cinema – although action films, in particular, seem to be directed in the opposite direction: a re-structuring of the *socius* through a reaffirmation and hardening of supposedly pre-existing structures projected into the subject to create the social body. In its affective dimension as an enveloping event, this reaffirmation follows the temporary threat of a deterritorialization of the subject into the body without organs as a renewal of superior male identity.

The crisis of the action image

However loosely defined, the action film as a genre relies more heavily on the movement-image (which entails the action, affection, and perception image) than on the time-image. In terms of the movement image, considering the film experience as an event entails two poles: on the one hand there is the sensory-motor scheme of the action image and on the other hand the purely optical and aural situation in which perception itself is what happens and what constitutes the cinematic event. While the perception image exists only to be seen and the spectators' sense of being there and seeing already exhausts the event's meaning, the action image relates to the sensory-motor schema of goal orientated and purposive action. What is called the 'crisis of the action image' follows directly from this relation between the action image and the sensory-motor schema of goal orientation and purposive action. Its crisis (that of the image but also of its relation to said schema) manifests itself in situations in which no action is possible anymore, effecting a rupture of the sensory-motor links. This loss of linkage is frequently compensated for in mainstream action films of the last two decades by a kind of psychotic hyperactivity, in which the movement and action come at the characters, rather than emanating from them. The consequences are either characters that exist only inside each others' minds, or an action scenario in which some thing, be it a natural world (as in *Twister* or *Volcano*), creature (as in the *Terminator* films), human (as in the *Die Hard* or *Rambo* films), or technology (as in the *Matrix* films) are out of control and the protagonists can re-act to them only by shielding themselves from being attacked or annihilated. Action in the fullest meaning of the word is no longer possible, and the action image reveals only an effort at blocking intensities, deflecting them to uphold existing structures. As my wording of the last sentence suggests, there is a fundamental parallel between the crisis of the action image and the subject's reaction to the productivity of pain in mainstream action films. Much like they deflect and shield themselves from their enemies' attacks, the male protagonists of these films also deflect the deterritorializing intensities threatening the organization of their social bodies until, at the limit of the deterritorialized flow, they approach the construction of a body without organs. While it would be sheer speculation to argue that either has brought forth the other, the two phenomena being statements produced by the same representational machines, it appears natural to assume an interrelationship between them – if only that these statements are necessarily desires and that, in the production of these statements, they contribute equally to an affirmation of the illusion of a fixed and stable subject.

Since the action image establishes a relationship between movement and actions, while the perception image establishes one between movement and bodies, Deleuze distinguishes two forms of the action image that can structure the narrative on a global or local level, one 'small', the other 'large'. The former posits an action (A), which leads to or encounters a situation (S), which in turn leads to a new form or kind of action (A'). In the latter, the beginning is a (more or less) stable situation (S), which leads to or encounters an action (A), which in turn causes a new situation (S'). While Deleuze discusses both the small and the large form of the action image on the same level in terms of narrative structure, I want to argue that the two can be interdependent and actually intermesh on different scales. More precisely, it seems that the large form of SAS' in the mainstream action films discussed here actually reveals an ASA' structure on a more detailed level. In this particular type of the small form we might designate the situation that exposes the protagonist to the productivity of pain as S^p, with the qualification that S^p is still part of the unchanged situation S in the global SAS' structure of the film narrative.

A reading which, on all levels, brings together and integrates a number of strands in Deleuze's work and thought thus yields a more detailed description of the particular action image under consideration here. It can account for the how, on a diegetic level, these films articulate the productivity of pain so as to conceal the deterritorializing effects of pain while foregrounding its indirect effect: the male hero's well-structured and socially productive identity in the form of the *socius*. This holds for most mainstream action films, regardless of whether pain becomes productive on the level of global narrative structure or merely on the level of one particular fight. In the former, the productivity of pain is extended considerably so that it can function as an organizing line of flight in the entire narrative, while in the latter, it works momentarily to produce a well-structured body facilitating the male character's always expected, yet always implausible victory against impossible odds. And while a deconstructive reading can open up mainstream action films to such a Deleuzean perspective on pain, these filmic events do not emphasize any of the lines of politics as defined by Deleuze and Guattari in *A Thousand Plateaus* and again by Deleuze in *Dialogues*, where he distinguishes between three political lines: the segmental line, the molecular line, and the line of flight. Like the lines of flight projected into the structured body of the male protagonists exposed to the productivity of pain, such lines of politics are deflected by these films so as to reaffirm the subject as a stable self in the service of society; it takes the work of deconstruction to unearth their directionality and reclaim the deterritorializing productivity of pain.

Works Cited

Ansell Pearson, Keith. *Germinal Life: The Difference and Repetition of Deleuze*. London: Routledge, 1999.

Bogue, Ronald. *Deleuze and Guattari*. London: Routledge, 1989.

Braidotti, Rosi. "Meta(l)morphoses." Featherstone 67–80.

Buchanan, Ian. *Deleuzism: A Metacommentary*. Durham, NC: Duke UP, 2000.

Deleuze, Gilles. *Cinema 1: The Movement Image*. Trans. Hugh Tomlinson and Barbara Habberjam. London: Athlone, 1986.

— *Spinoza: Practical Philosophy*. Trans. Robert Hurley. San Francisco: City Lights, 1987.

— *Cinema 2: The Time Image*. Trans. Hugh Tomlinson & Robert Galeta. London: Athlone, 1989.

— *The Logic of Sense*. Trans. Mark Lester. London: Athlone, 1999.

— "Dualism, Monism and Multiplicities: Desire – Pleasure – Jouissance. Seminar of 26 March 1973." Trans. Daniel W. Smith. *Contretemps* 2 (May 2001): 92–108.

— and Claire Parnet. *Dialogues*. Trans. Hugh Tomlinson and Barbara Habberjam. London: Athlone, 1987.

— and Felix Guattari. *Anti-Oedipus. Capitalism and Schizophrenia*. Trans. Helen R. Lane and Robert Hurley. Minneapolis: U of Minnesota P, 1985.

— *A Thousand Plateaus. Capitalism and Schizophrenia*. Trans. Brian Massumi. London: Athlone, 1987.

Elsaesser, Thomas and Warren Buckland. *Studying Contemporary American Film: A Guide to Movie Analysis*. London: Arnold, 2002.

Featherstone, Mike, ed. *Gilles Deleuze: A Symposium*. Special Issue of *Theory, Culture and Society* 14. 2 (May 1997).

Foucault, Michel. "Theatrum Philosophicum." *Language, Counter-Memory, Practice. Selected Essays and Interviews*. Ed. Donald F. Bouchard. Trans. Donald F. Bouchard and Sherry Simon. Ithaca: Cornell UP, 1977. 165–96.

Grossberg, Lawrence. *Bringing It All Back Home: Essays on Cultural Studies*. Durham: Duke UP, 1997.

— *Dancing in Spite of Myself: Essays on Popular Culture*. Durham: Duke UP, 1997.

Millet, Nick. "The Trick of Singularity." Featherstone 50–68.

Morrell, David. "Writer's Commentary." *Rambo: First Blood. Special Edition DVD*, 2003.

Pisters, Patricia. "The Possibilities of Immanence." *Film-Philosophy* 3. 14 (March 1999) <http://www.film-philosophy.com/vol3-1999/n14pisters>.

— ed. *Micropolitics of Media Culture: Reading the Rhizomes of Deleuze and Guattari*. Amsterdam: Amsterdam UP, 2001.

Storey, John. "The Articulation of Memory and Desire: From Vietnam to the War in the Persian Gulf." *Memory and Popular Film*. Ed. Paul Grainge. Manchester: Manchester UP, 2003. 82–101.

Surin, Kenneth. "The 'Epochality' of Deleuzean Thought." Featherstone 9–21.

Femina Monstruosa. Femininity as Trauma in Robinson Jeffers' *Medea* and George Tabori's *M*

Isabel Capeloa Gil
Universidade Católica Portuguesa

1. Preamble or *corpo-realities*

Western culture rests upon a set of norms which are intrinsically prescriptive. Deviants, by lack or excess, have been clearly and sharply excluded from the community and the normative body politic from the beginnings of human history. In the Bible, Leviticus 21 tells us about the banishment from God's presence of those who are disabled or physically 'blemished':

> Whosoever he be of thy seed in their generations that hath any blemish, let him not approach to offer the bread of his God.
> For whatsoever man he be that hath a blemish, he shall not approach: a blind man, or a lame, or he that hath a flat nose, or anything superfluous,
> Or a man that is brokenfooted, or brokenhanded,
> Or crookback, or a dwarf or that hath a blemish in his eye, or be scurvy, or scabbed, or hath his stones broken. (L, 21, 17–20)

Studying this quote with greater detail reveals that Leviticus banishes from God's presence all those with 'blemishes'. This is a rather vague but very comprehensive term, as it refers to all those situated outside the 'zero degree of monstrosity', be it in biological, anthropological or racial terms. The author of the text then proceeds to define some of these blemishes, characterized by default (a lame or a blind man) or excess ('he that hath [...] anything superfluous'). Although able to participate in the glory of the law, bread of the Lord, anyone marked with a 'blemish' is excluded from His presence. In this archaic biblical configuration the one outside the norm, deviant by lack or excess, is displaced from the religious community, which affirms its own identity through his exclusion. Something else this biblical passage tells us is that the norm is not essential but contingent, i. e., depending on the substantive situation of that or those who posit themselves as the norm.

Literature, both in its dimension as a body of text *(corpus)* and as a representation of the body, tends to conform to dual concepts of the 'conquered' (Virilio 5), disciplined, prescribed body, constructed as performance in the intersection of normative, disciplinary and power discourses, versus the 'volatile' (Grosz 2), provisory one that tries to evade normalisation (e. g., in dance and performance-art).[1] The textual body is configured through the circulation of aesthetic energies which are culture founding and culture receptive and is thus representative of the inscription as incision of phallogocentric cultural norms. The process is by no means only one-way, but rather results from intertwined performative affirmative, i. e., normalising, and subversive procedures. It is from this dichotomous process that body identity and subject identity arise, are confirmed and restated. As Butler (154), Braidotti (82) and de Lauretis (120) have argued, this procedure is eventually constructed in relation to the norm, which is male, white, young, Western and physically fit, i. e., showing a zero degree of deviation.

Stemming from this understanding, my purpose in this paper is to show how literature/culture deals with deviant figura-

1 The radical experimentation with the material possibilities of the body is a trend in contemporary performance-art, particularly that of Meg Stuart or Marina Abramovic.

tions in sexual, racial and physical terms.[2] My subject-matter, Medea, is the absolute embodiment of deviation and monstrosity. As a woman, she represents the realm of the 'other-than' the norm, be it in terms of excess or lack. Woman is the enigma – in Freudian terms –, a displaced entity existing outside the norm that still depends on her and on her sacrifice for its own existence, as argued by Elisabeth Bronfen:

> Woman comes to represent the margins or extremes of the norm – the extremely good, pure and helpless, or the extremely dangerous, chaotic and seductive [...]. As the outsider per se, woman can also come to stand for a complete negation of the ruling norm, for the element which disrupts the bounds of normal conventions and the passage through which that threat to the norm is articulated [...]. Over her dead body, cultural norms are reconfirmed or secured, whether because the sacrifice of the virtuous, innocent woman serves a social critique and transformation or because a sacrifice of the dangerous woman re-establishes an order that was momentarily suspended due to her presence. (181)

Medea represents the absolute Other, the Other-within culture – the woman – as well as the Other-without, the Other culture, inscribed in the colour of her skin, in her deviant cultural practices, in her irrationality, exoticism, as well as in her knowledge of sorcery. The Otherness is enhanced by her disruption of the maternal figure, thus well embodying the simultaneous awe, fascination and abjection felt by man before the feminine maternal body (Braidotti 79 ff.). As life-giving and death-announcing, the mother's body functions as an eternal traumatic remembrance of man's ephemeral existence, functioning both as culture-founding and culture-disruptive. Medea's myth further discusses the way in which culture deals with the prospect of its own bodily and spiritual annihilation.

2 Figuration is used here both in the sense of a representation of situated knowledges in terms of race, age, sex, religion and geography, as Donna Haraway has argued (12), as well as an aesthetic figure perceived throughout the threads of the text, as in Paul de Man's definition (25).

My purpose is thus to discuss both the transgressive appeal and the empowerment mode of trauma and pain that this mythical story has exerted upon much of Western imagination, by focussing on two figurations of the myth in drama: Robinson Jeffers' *Medea* (1946) and George Tabori's *M* (1984).[3] These two plays are representative of dichotomous ways of coming to terms with Medea; the former by pursuing an affirmative reception of the traditional story and portraying disruption as indeed culture-founding; the latter by subverting the myth and tradition and creating a simulacrum of Medea.[4] Moreover, the play co-opts the heroine, thus transferring the Otherness to the norm, to the Father and the way he deals with the disabled son.

2. The woman as monster *(femina monstruosa)*

In her book *Nomadic Subjects*, Rosi Braidotti writes that 'the monstrous as the negative pole, the pole of pejoration, is structurally analogous to the feminine as that which is other than the established norm' (80). Medea is the *femina monstruosa* in that she subsumes the radical Otherness of the woman with the deviation, by lack or excess, of the monstrous.

3 All quotes from Jeffers' play shall be referred to as JM, and from Tabori's text quotations shall be signaled TM.

4 These two texts are examples of what I may call, with Lisa Lowe, the 'heterotopicality' of discourses about Medea. She writes: 'Discourses are heterogeneously and irregularly composed of statements and restatements, contentions and accommodation, generated by a plurality of writing positions at any given moment [...]. In other words, the use of the notion of a dominant discourse is incomplete if not accompanied by a critique which explains why some positions are easily co-opted and integrated into apparently-dominant discourses, and why others are less likely to be appropriated' (236).

According to the *Oxford Dictionary of English*, the monster is defined as that which is 'abnormally misshapen; an imaginary creature or person remarkable for some bad or evil quality'. This definition covers bodily deviation and moral debasement as well as its exclusion from real existence, by branding it imaginary. Another trait of the monster is its unnaturalness.[5] The monster jeopardizes and disrupts the order of nature, its configuration is either a sign of the aberration of the natural order or, much worse than that, the statement that there is no order. On the other hand, the monster is also the fascinating Other, both seductive and threatening in its difference, embodied with a destabilising force that disrupts the self's identity. With its ambivalence and powerful disruptive force, the monster is positioned beyond, before and after the norm, it lurks in that blank space of indefinition, waiting to be activated in order to confirm the positivity of the norm.

In teratology, the science of monsters devised by Geoffroy Saint-Hillaire in the 19th century, the monster is defined in terms of excess, lack or displacement of organs. First, there is a striking likeness between this physical symptomatology and the way woman is defined in relation to the male-cultural norm. Woman is excessive, both sexually, as the sexually hyperactive *femme fatale*; as well as politically, due to her transgression of the established norms. Second, she is also defined through lack; lack of masculinity, or lack of the phallus as Lacan argued (687), or also as lacking substantial subjective unity, she is 'the sex which is not

5 Rosi Braidotti analyses Ambroise Paré's treaty *Des monstres et prodigs*, Geneva 1573, and discusses the evolution of the concept of monstrosity since Antiquity, arguing that only relatively late in human history, particularly in the 19th century, did monsters start to be perceived as human freaks, as conceived by man and woman in a procedure that went wrong (88). In Antiquity, monsters were seen as being of divine or non-human origin. Woman was, according to Aristotle in the *Generation of Animals*, the only freak of nature, as conceived only when something other than the norm happened in the reproductive process.

one', in Luce Irigaray's ironic assertion (1). Third, woman is the embodiment of displacement in that she is the 'other-than', existing beyond boundaries, like a nomad walking the margins. As the *khôra* of culture (Kristeva 35), woman is a 'becoming-metaphor' (Braidotti 83). She has no place in culture, but it depends on her for its definition of placement. In physical terms, the female body is also transgressive in that it has no absolute shape, it is morphed by pregnancy to absorb and envelop another body. It swells, grows; it is indeed a volatile body, in a never-ceasing metamorphosis that is thereafter endangering to the male norm as it is from this 'monstrous' origin that he himself descends.

The mingling of abjection and awe is a *topos* in the configuration of the mother's body. It is simultaneously hellish and holy, repulsive and fascinating, dirty and pure (Douglas 234), placed on the threshold between the human and the divine creation effort. It is therefore no wonder, despite the tautology of the definition *femina monstruosa*, that a mother, and in fact a murderous mother may come to represent the absolute monstrosity of the feminine, both in its greatness, violence and disruption as well as in the embodiment of woman's abuse by the phallogocentric order.

3. Medea/ M/ Monster/ Man/ Myth

I shall start by the last signifier: Myth. As narrative structures, myths provide aesthetic configurations which convey a certain form of 'world readability' ('Lesbarkeit der Welt') (Blumenberg 25). They have a parabolic framework (Fühmann 206) which, though contradictory, has been useful in figuring social aporias, psychic situations, identity problems and power relations. The productiveness of mythic categories has been confirmed in every aesthetic medium, ranging from painting, sculpture, literature, music and dance to theatre, opera and performance art. Of those myths stemming from the Greek-Roman world, the story of Medea, though one of the most violent, has undoubtedly been one of the most productive.[6]

Despite the statement by Ranke Graves that the Euripidean constellation of the mythical story, portraying Medea as a barbaric sorceress, is not true, this construct has become a *topos* in Western culture. Ranke Graves (167) and other renowned classicists such as Karl Kerényi (20) or Kurt von Fritz (332) challenge the Euripidean configuration. They regard Medea rather as a goddess from Colchis in the Caucasus or as a founding-heroine (Krevans 71 & Johnston 45). The divine characteristics of the heroine which have been maintained in Euripides' tragedy, portraying her as the granddaughter of Helios, the Sun, account for her escape in a chariot pulled by serpents. The relation of the myth to Moon goddesses such as Hecate has been analysed by Johannes Gascard, who argues that the character was originally called *Bona Dea*, a Moon divinity, protectress of childbirth, but took up the name *Medea* as Jason's lover and thus acquired more human characteristics (145). Again according to Ranke Graves, the Corinthians had

6 Let us recall after Euripides' tragedy, *Medea* (431 BC), Seneca's *Medea*, Corneille's *Medée* (1635), F. M. Klinger's, *Medea in Corinth* (1787) and *Medea auf dem Kaukasus* (1791) Grillparzer's, *Das goldene Vließ* (1821), Hans Henny Jahnn's *Medea* (1920), Corrado Alvaro's *Lunga Notte di Medea* (1949), Pier Paolo Pasolini's *Medea*, Heiner Müllers, *Volkommenes Ufer. Medeamaterial. Landschaft mit Argonauten* (1983), and more recently Ursula Haas' novel, *Freispruch für Medea* as well as Christa Wolf's *Medea. Stimmen* (1996). In music, one may mention the operas *Thesée* by Quinault/Lulli (1675), *Medea* by Cherubini (1797), Ernst Krenek's *Der goldene Bock* (1964) and recently Rolf Liebermann's *Medea* (1994). Medea has also inspired a number of painters, particularly in the Modern Age, such as the Pre-Raphaelite Frederick Sandys (1866–68), Anselm Feuerbach with *Medea und die Urne* (1870), or Anselm Kiefer's *Die Argonautent* (1990). In dance, American Martha Graham has also performed a choreography on the Medea saga entitled *Cave of the Heart* (1946).

done her wrong by banishing her from the city, and in compensation, they would have paid Euripides to portray the story in a fashion which would spare them guilt and bad reputation (12ff.).

No matter what classical philology or anthropology tells us, the fact is that this reappraisal of the myth has stimulated limited cultural productivity in recent years, for instance in Christa Wolf's novel, *Medea Stimmen* (1996) or in *M* by George Tabori. Both configurations are representative of the inversion of Medea's role from the assassin or the monster to the victim. Medea is coopted by political correctness and experiences a shift from one male-centered defilement to a victimized debasement.

In the development of European culture, Medea has come to embody the gendered Western Orientalist discourse. The eccentric subjectivity of Medea, posited both as an Asian barbarian from the Caucasus, i. e., geographically peripheral to the Greek (read Western) centre, as well as a woman, i. e., displaced from the normativity of the *polis*, and from citizenship, has moreover been inscribed with the markings of radical racial Otherness in the colonialist discourse. Despite the geographical location of Colchis, she is usually represented as a black woman, so as to enhance both her physical and moral strangeness and stress her deviation from normative whiteness. The whole construction of the myth is based on what Said calls the set of polarities which divide the West and the Rest (21). She is therefore marked out as exotic, irrational, erotic, despotic and heathen (Lewis 18), and figures as a synecdoche *per se* of the Orient, very often portrayed pejoratively as feminine in racist discourses.

The sexually hyperactive *femme fatale*, the irrational sorceress, who dismembers and disrupts in order to grant Jason power, the ethnical Other, but also the former powerful princess, is in fact a projection of male civilized fears. The dread of the Other-without is embodied in the distorted vision of the Other-within, thus justifying both external, imperialistic and colonial disciplinary measures as well as internal ones, subsumed in the normalisation of Medea by the Corinthian *ethos*.

Medea's path is that of a failed socialization. The Argonaut saga of Apollonius of Rhodes and Euripides tells us about courage, honour, violence, but only exerted for the greatness of the Greek male hero, Jason. His allure is so great that he converts and seduces the barbarian Medea who, by conforming to the role of the mother and by submitting to Jason's patriarchal order, begins the path of subjugation debated in Euripides' tragedy:

> Surely, of all creatures that have life and will, we women
> Are the most wretched. When for an extravagant sum,
> We have bought a husband, we must then accept him as
> Possessor of our body. This is to aggravate
> Wrong with worse wrong.Then the great question: will the man
> We get be bad or good? For women, divorce is not
> Respectable; to repel the man, not possible.
>
> Still more, a foreign woman, coming among new laws,
> New customs, needs the skill of magic, to find out
> What her home could not teach her, how to treat the man
> Whose bed she shares. And if in this exacting toil
> We are successful, and our husband does not struggle
> Under the marriage yoke, our life is enviable.
> Otherwise death is better. (228–41)

Medea acknowledges bodily submission to her husband and submits to the order of the city. However, her spirit brings forth a knowledge unsubjugated by the order of reason. The disruptive potential lurking beneath the ordered surface of Greek regulatory practices comes forth in an orgy of violence, murder and revenge. Thus, the disruptive and violent acts committed at the core of the myth in order to steal the Golden Fleece from Colchis are reenacted. Let us recall the dismembering of Medea's brother, Absyrtus, or the dismembering of Jason's treacherous uncle, Pelias. These disruptive actions are ritually repeated in Medea's sacrifice of the boys, representing the monstrosity lying behind normativity and patterning cultural evolution to a model of violence which hides the prospect of its own annihilation. Medea's story is a rightful representation of how the body as colony strikes back.

I shall now turn to the other signifiers in the subtitle 'Medea/ M/ Monster/ Man' through the discussion of Robinson Jeffers' *Medea* and George Tabori's *M*, examples of remarkable power shifts in the appreciation of dominant cultural discourses. The approach to these plays shows the heterotopicality that a discourse perceived as phallogocentric, imperial and prescriptive has acquired in the 20th century, having for centuries formed the discussion around Medea. As I referred earlier, these are two opposite approaches to the same myth. Although both deal with transgression, Jeffers does it in an affirmative way, using transgression as legitimisation of order and inscribed in the power structures that portray Medea as the *femina monstruosa*. Tabori creates a simulated Medea, which he calls *M*. Medea as the lack of herself is reduced to M, a subversion of tradition, but also a subversion of culture and its strategies.

Robinson Jeffers' *Medea*, written in 1946, opened on Broadway to enthusiastic reviews in October 1947[7] with Judith Anderson in the title role and John Gielgud, who also directed the play, as Jason. Strangely enough, though Jeffers was long considered an outcast (Vardamis 60) who focussed most of his writing on poetry, it is for *Medea* and another dramatic poem, *Cawdor* (the American story of Theseus and Phaedra) that he acquired more

7 In a review dated 21 October 1947, Brooks Atkinson of the *New York Times* called this play a landmark of the modern stage (in Karman 153). Kappo Phelan stressed the barbarism of Anderson's interpretation (154). This enthusiasm to which Anderson's performance no doubt contributed contrasts with the book reviews that appeared in 1946, such as in the *York Times Book Review* on 21 April 1946 by Donald A. Stauffer, called 'California Euripides', where the critic says the work is 'neither a great tragedy nor a good poem. It is a melodrama that falls between the two styles' (152). The same detachment from great drama is enhanced in a review written by Lisle Bell, appearing on 21 April 1946 in the *Weekly Book Review*, stating that '[T]he reader of this version will not sense the operatic nature of Greek tragedy, but he will feel without question its tremendous dramatic impact' (19). For other criticism see Boswell, 60–66.

notoriety. This play, written specially for actress Judith Anderson, a friend of the Jeffers family, was of particular interest to Jeffers, due to what his wife Una called his identification with Euripides (Karman 135), prompted by his loneliness, and the antagonism to war and violence expressed in his plays.[8] In fact, as Alex Vardamis argues, Jeffers, a poet who retreated from society to build a lonely stone tower at Point Sur, on the California coast, has rarely been judged on the merits of his poetry alone: 'Accused of fascism, communism, anarchism, pacifism, isolationism, sadism, misanthropy and atheism, he remains a poet of great power' (44).

Whether *Medea* represented 'the hate-filled violence of a war that had just claimed millions of innocent lives' (Karman 137), or an ecological revenge of nature embodied in the woman Medea (Hesse 141), or even the psychological malaise of a sick civilization (Brophy 171), Jeffers' heroine is undoubtedly an extraordinary

8 By substituting Greece for Western civilization and Athens for America, Jeffers positions himself as an 'America first' defender, further enhanced by his identification with Euripides during the World War II period: 'There were other counts against Euripides. His great precursors were more than poets and playwrights; they were also exemplary citizens [...]. But Euripides remained a private man, a disillusioned student and man of letters. The world had changed in his time, the great dream was fading. Recently Athens had been the saviour of all Greece; but now Greece had fallen apart, and Athens, though grown much greater, was only an imperialistic power struggling with Sparta for supremacy, busy with confused battles and oppressions. Therefore, as many honest men have done since his time, Euripides chose to stay aloof from private life; and it seems to me that he was right in his time; but his fellow-citizens judged otherwise' (in Bennet 217). Jeffers' criticism of the American participation in World War II came from having witnessed the horror and trauma of World War I. This posture can be seen particularly in the poetry volume *Be Angry at the Sun* (1941), as well as in *The Double Axe and Other Poems*, published in 1948, which contained political views that made the editor, Random House, disclaim responsibility for the contents in the preface added to the book. One instance that caused a political stir was his naming of Hitler, Churchill, Roosevelt and Stalin as warlords. Jeffers' isolationism was almost universally condemned in the post-war years.

regressive, primeval being, drunk with violence and death wishes, the very embodiment of a dawning cultural apocalypse.

Reverting to the archaic geographic origins of the myth, Jeffers casts Medea as Asian (JM 117). Though this is a departure from the black-other-model that many twentieth century Medeas have embodied, Jeffers' Asian woman has, in the context of the American post-war years, an even more radical Otherness. The Asian enemy, the Asian fiend, a projection of the war suffering in East Asia assumes a monstrous materiality in this Medea.

Here we are faced with a universe from which ideals have disappeared, leaving behind wounded and injured bodies. Mankind is depicted as a suffering body, marked from its outset with grief, where even the life drives, such as love, 'walk in blood' (JM 141). Existence is only possible in blood, violence and death, and discourse is constructed as what Dietmar Kamper calls a 'scarred writing' ('Narbenschrift') (1–7), showing the textual bodies of the characters as surfaces written by pain. In fact, there is no place for humanism in this play, or for humanity for that matter.

While Jason and Creon represent the rational, subjugated knowledge, the norm and the power in the play, their self-centredness, egotism, greed and the cold Greek rational logic prove to be totally vulnerable to the excluded Otherness they try to dominate. Not only are they bad judges of character, misinterpreting Medea's words, but they also fall prey to her submissive strategy when sending the children with deadly gifts for Jason's new bride, Creüsa. Despite the fact that she is a woman and a foreigner, the all-enveloping cosmopolitan Greek democratic discourse views Medea as 'dominable'. The norm is so limited and helpless in its prescriptiveness that it does not know how to deal with the Other within and without itself, and also, due to the imposition of universality, bears within itself the seeds of its own disruption.

Medea, Jason's helper, was a man's instrument of power, representing the hideous Other within the Self for the male-centred power construct. Jason is only Jason because Medea helped him in the robbery of the Golden Fleece. Medea's banishment releases the monstrous Other from the rationality of the Self. She must therefore be depicted as Other and outside mankind. From her topical nomadic locations as a foreigner, barbarian, sorceress and woman, Jeffers' Medea is debased in the chain of being. First, she is denied humanity by being depicted with an animal-like body language. She 'moves like a caged animal' (JM 119), describes the sacrifice of the children as something that 'glares in my eyes / Like a lion on a ridge' (JM 180), while the word used by the eldest child running away from her is 'she is hunting me' (JM 184). Then Jason names her 'a beast, like a crawling viper' (JM 188). Yet he recognizes the mistake of this classification when after the murder of the children he says 'No wild beast could have done it' (JM 189). Medea is not an animal. Her excess outweighs configurations within the animal realm.

Then Medea is portrayed as a Medusa-character, and defiled into a mineral. She has hostile eyes (JM 121), she is a stone with stone eyes (JM 114), 'rigid with inner violence' (JM 136), and is addressed by Creon as 'woman of the stone forehead and hate-filled eyes' (JM 124). Medea is the object of the male-appalled gaze of the Other, and the subject of a gaze that embodies the dread of petrifaction, either of Man or/and culture.

However, these inscriptions are somehow different than those self-ascribed by Medea, and here lies perhaps the greatest challenge in the play. Medea does not self-construct herself as a monster, but she conforms to the situation of the one which is other-than the norm. She places herself as the ethnic outsider and excuses her racial Otherness with humanity, she speaks with the voice of the Western dominant subject, inscribing her racial markings as inferior *vis-à-vis* Creüsa's whiteness, whose attributes she uses to beg Creon's pardon: 'I beseech you / By the soft yellow hair and cool smooth forehead and the white knees /of that young girl' (JM 130). Creusa represents the zero degree of Otherness, she embodies in Adrienne Rich's words, the 'thoughtless whiteness' (219) of the race with no markings. She is white, blond and young, sharply contrasted to Medea, the middle-aged foreigner, an Asian virago.

When lamenting her situation, that of a woman banished by her husband, Medea hesitates in her own self-assessment: 'I do not know what other women [...]. I do not know how much a Greek woman/ will endure. The people of my race are somewhat rash and intemperate [...]. As for me I simply want to die' (JM 122). Medea places herself both outside the ethnical and the anthropological norms. She is not just a woman, and she is not Greek, therefore she does not know what a Greek woman may endure. She posits herself in the ambivalent position of woman as culture operative and as culture subversive, acting both inside and outside the norm, which makes her even more dangerous as that which has no place, no denomination and is not subjugated to any order of discourse.

The sacrifice of the children is also a sign of this total ambivalence, which finds its absolute representation in death, and Medea has been the very embodiment of death from the beginning. Her first line is rather an anticipation of her role in the whole economy of the play: 'Death. Death is my wish. For myself, my enemies, my children. Destruction/ That's the word. Grind, crush, burn. Destruction' (JM 117). She becomes Eris the destroyer and is secured in the position of the outcast murderess. Let us recall that at this stage, Medea's path is marked by murder, that of Absyrtus, her brother, and Pelias, Jason's uncle. They are killed and dismembered, Absyrtus' body parts thrown at those persecuting the Argonauts, Pelias is dismembered by his daughters believing they would thus rejuvenate him. Both deaths function as the founding violence that stands for evolution and change. The dismembering of Absyrtus' body, though a strategy to slow down the Argo's persecutors, recalls the sacrifice of the young king or of the young God, as can be ritually observed in the rituals of Adonis or those of Osiris in Egypt. Frazer (225ff.) and Assmann (44–79) argue that these rituals were performed to exercise the rejuvenation of the community, symbolically embodied in re-membering the body during the Spring rituals. As for Pelias, his dismembering functions as a parody of that same ritual, but renewal also arises in the figure of Jason, the new king.

What the foreground of the Medea story tells us is that evolution and change, even in a 'civilised' world, submit to the ritual principles of violence and sacrifice, which as Girard tells us will be mimetized throughout the course of the community's history (12) in order to re-legitimise its existence. The fact that in rational Greece, distanced from 'the dirt and superstition of Asiatic Colchis' (JM 139) these founding rites were not observed as legitimate, religiously sanctioned violence but as disruptive acts, amounts to the inability of normalised societies to deal with the disruption at its core. Medea's agency of murder excludes her from the community of civilised women and men, so that the prohibitions and regulations applied to these lack bearing on her actions. This is also true of the 'natural' prohibition of infanticide.

The chorus of women expresses this regulation as a natural truth: 'Women hate war, but men will wage it again./ Women may hate their husbands, and sons their fathers,/ But women will never hate their own children' (JM 143). These lines express relations between the sexes as war, the relationship between sons and fathers as agonistic and utters a 'normalised' law of nature, namely that women will never hurt their children. This is a sign of the 'machinery of institutional violence wrenching at the experience of motherhood' (Rich 280), and therefore the revolt against the institution could not find a more suitable and radical example as in the denial and subversion of this taboo.

The fact that infanticide is not just murder *per se* can be observed in the formulation used by Medea in her appearance before Aegeus, king of Athens. While begging for asylum, she asks how he would take revenge on his enemy, and he answers the first thing would be to kill his progeny, for through his progeny the enemy's existence prevails after death. Medea then comments remarkably 'Unchild him, ha?/And then unlife him.' (JM 146) This line marks a turning point in the play. Observe that Medea does not use the signifier 'kill', meaning a violent end to an existing being, but rather denies the very existence of the children and Jason's by using the prefix [un], 'unchild', 'unlife'. Medea's purpose is now far more devious than at the beginning of the play, she no longer lusts for 'mere' death, but for un-existence, materialized in the wiping out of memory, the real forum for perennial existence. The beheading of the children is the last step in a process of dissolution and dismembering, a radical ending to the notion of dismembering as sacrifice which the aforementioned deaths of Absyrtus and Pelias represent.

The banishment as traumatic event has caused in Medea an understanding of existence, past, present and future as inscribed by the markings of pain. The productivity of pain as the founding element of the *memoria*, which underlies the very permanence of culture can be traced back to Nietzsche, who in the *Genealogie der Moral* argues that:

> Es gibt vielleicht nichts furchtbarer und unheimlicher an der ganzen Vorgeschichte des Menschen, als seine *Mnemotechnik*. 'Man brennt etwas ein, damit es im Gedächtnis bleibt: nur was nicht aufhört, *wehzutun*, bleibt im Gedächtnis' – das ist ein Hauptsatz aus der ältesten (leider auch allerlängsten) Psychologie auf Erden [...]. Es ging niemals ohne Blut, Martern, Opfer ab, wenn den Mensch es nötig hielt, sich ein Gedächtnis zu machen. (209)

Pain is a mnemonic inscription on the body, the marking that underlies every form of representation. The traumatic experience of banishment, seen as a symbolical dismembering of Medea from the community's body,[9] prompts a disruption marked at the language level by the obsession of radicalizing this exclusion. The trauma is well embodied in the following lines:

9 The notion of community as body stems from Paul, who in Ephesians 4, 13–16, intertwines the body of Christ with the community of Christians. On the notion of community as a body see Kantorowicz, 20ff and Foucault 27–35.

> This is it. I did not surely know it: loathing is all. This flesh
> He has touched and fouled. These hands that wrought for him, these knees
> That ran his errands. This body that took his ... what they call love,
> and made children of it. If I could peel off
> The flesh, the children, the memory...
> Poor misused hand: poor defiled arm: your bones
> Are not unshapely. If I could tear off the flesh and be bones;
> naked bones
> Salt-scoured bones on the shore
> At home in Colchis. (JM 141)

The path of dis-membering as a form of dis-membrance then moves from the form of self-dismembering that the language materializes, and represents her drifting, self- and hetero-exclusion from the Greek community, to the disruption of the community itself, embodied in the king, Creon and his daughter. The death by poison and holocaust is described in images of dissolution that drive language to the limits of self-disruption:

> NURSE: [...] that doomed girl
> Frightfully crying started up from the chair; she ran, she was
> like
> a torch, and the gold crown
> Like a comet streamed fire; she tore at it but it clung to her
> head;
> the golden cloak
> Was white-hot, flaying the flesh from the living bones; blood
> mixed with fire ran down, she fell, she burned
> On the floor, writhing. Then Creon came and flung himself
> on her, hoping to choke
> That rage of flame, but it ran through him, his own agony
> Made him forget his daughter's. The fire stuck to the flesh,
> it glued him to her; he tried to stand up,
> He tore her body and his own. The burnt flesh broke
> In lumps from the bones. [...]
> They lie there.
> Eyeless, disfaced, untouchable; middens of smoking flesh
> laced
> with molten gold. (JM179)

In an incredible orgy of dissolution, Medea dismembers the powers that excluded and displaced her and then moves to disband and destroy her own contribution for the existence of the community. By killing her children, she is displaced from her last position in the cultural order, as a mother, and definitely shifts into the monstrous position of the excessive non-human, evil god-like sorceress who elopes in the Sun's chariot with the small corpses. This action is pursued so that in the representational sphere no *ars memoriativa*, as a physical form of perennial memory, is left of them. The effacement of memory, as the most disruptive of acts, is nevertheless contradicted by Jeffers' textual strategy, which leaves Jason and the *corpus* as the textual body of the play, as re-membering instruments, re-membering bodies. This is uttered by the escaping Medea's proleptic discourse announcing Jason's degrading and dismembered death under the rotting timber of the Argos: '[...] meanwhile sit there/ and mourn, remembering the infinite evil, and the good/ That has turned evil' (JM 190). It is ultimately a statement that in man, culture – like memory – lives on.

On the opposite side of this representation of Medea lies George Tabori's *M* (1984), an exercise of myth subversion and a politically correct rewriting of Euripides, which opened in the Münchner Kammerspiele on 3 January 1985. This Jewish, Hungarian-born British citizen (1914), playwright who works in Austria, is himself an example of displacement and his theatre is particularly characterized by his apology of victims, the call against tyranny and oppression, war and violence. Tabori is more widely known for his holocaust theatre, specially such plays as *The Cannibals* or *Mein Kampf*, where he debates the issue of violence from the very personal experience of his family's annihilation in Auschwitz. Tabori's interest in the Medea story stems from what he believes is the need to end the old lies about Medea (Fischbach 301), pronouncing her innocent according to the verdicts of Ranke-Graves and Kerényi (TM 1). The effort to displace Medea as a screen for the projection of archaic-psychological male fears, as the representation of female evil, excess and monstrosity is accompanied by an investigation into the structure of normality itself, the structure of the male, logical, white, harmonious norm. The issue at stake is in fact vulnerability, the vulnerability of the weak before the dominant power structure, and he does this through two examples of extreme woundability, the slandered, manipulated and abused woman and the disabled child.

Tabori reduces the constellation of the myth to the primary family triangle, Man, Woman, Child. The excessive, and in that sense, the monstrous is no longer the ethnically strange woman, but rather the disabled, crippled child, who can only move in a wheelchair. The mother's attachment to the Child is starkly contrasted to the father's disgust, who sees his masculinity and his power over the Woman challenged by the malformed being. It is therefore he who kills the child and then tries to shift the guilt to the mother, Medea, that traditionally monstrous being who is capable of the utmost violence.

The Man tries to burden the Woman with the guilt of the Child's death through a number of devices, for instance, by manipulating a tape where she is speaking to Aegeus about his impotence problems. As in a play within the play, the Man presents himself as the theatrical director of the events that are about to unfold and orders the Child to act out the part of Medea in Euripides (TM 14). Peter Radtke, the actor cast with the role of the Child, a physically challenged actor with a sort of brittle bones disease, embodies the physical monstrosity and uses part of a 'disability play' called *News from Grottenholm* (*Nachricht vom Grottenholm*) (1980), to show the way in which society deals with deviation. The helpless disabled Child and the helpless Medea, two examples of deviation in the cultural order, are co-opted, i. e., normalized, by Tabori's theatre and made to represent a new order. In a scene with tremendous impact, in fact an intertextual quote of Radtke's aforementioned play, the Child and the Woman play the brotherhood of victims in an aggressor society:

WOMAN: Honey! Look at me! We are all crippled..
CHILD: We are not all crippled!
WOMAN: Yes, we are!
CHILD: Then look at me! Would you like to switch places with me?
WOMAN: Yes, froggy. (Radtke 115–16)

The Child bares his breast in a fashion that unveils the bone's malformation, showing him as a sort of freak of nature and revealing the mother's attention and care towards the vulnerable Child. Tabori plays upon cultural and body prescriptive taboos, positing them out as culturally and male power dependent to then uproot the monstrous deviation beneath the surface of normality. The issue is no longer the legitimisation of the community, or the showing of freakiness as norm-founding, but rather the confrontation of the normal as monstrous: in fact, the de-construction of the regulated, established norm.

It is here that Tabori's holocaust experience comes to the fore. In an interview published in the German newspaper, *Süddeutsche Zeitung* on 26 December 1984, Tabori draws on the recent experience of Fruchtmann's film on the Majdanek-Case, where the defendants – the guards and SS personnel – looked as normal and familiar as the victims. The witnesses were amazed at the normality of the monstrous aggressors, but in fact they had the wrong idea about the rule of normality. Tabori then adds that our history begins with murder and never stops using it. In fact, Auschwitz becomes a normal event within the path of devious behaviour (in Fischer 125).

Tabori's *M* disrupts the boundaries between normality and monstrosity, de-figuring the norm and dis-simulating it. The holocaust, or a child's murder, is equivalent in the scale of normal monstrosity. No longer the displaced Other, but now the regulated Self, the Man kills the Child, both in an attempt to control what is strange and Other to himself and as a strategy to reaffirm his position before the Woman. The Man's last lines represent the vulnerability of the weak, falling prey to the strong, but also Man's regressive behaviour, his narcissistic inability to distance himself from the imaginary, linked to the mother, and his longing for absolute dedication:

> It is always the children
> That are murdered,
> Thrown out of cliffs,
> Nailed to crosses,
> Slaughtered in wars,
> Killed before
> They kill the gods
> Here too, this is how it happened
> Hold me tight.
> Now, we are alone, as in the beginning
> In the circle of love
> Before he came
> And broke the bond.
> I always wanted to be the only one. (TM 35)

And so I end with a remark on the beginning. Tabori misreads Medea in order to re-figure the myth. He rehabilitates Euripides' victim and thus creates a copy which enacts the original through its presence in absence. We are faced with what Baudrillard calls a simulacrum (Baudrillard 14), a fake Medea who through repetition in reverse, marks the emptiness of the original. *M* is Medea, but also an appropriation of the title of the film *M* by Fritz Lang, which also dwells on a child's murder. In Tabori's own words: 'Well, M. What comes to your mind? Mother, murder, man, Medea, miscarriage, mythology, Munich. And then there is the film by Fritz Lang.' (in Fischer 125) As a simulated *Medea*, Tabori's drama shows the crisis in the representation of the myth, the operational shift in contemporary culture which can no longer find a suitable place for the disruption confirming the norm within the aporetic construction of displacement itself. Medea is no longer monstrous, she is a victim. M is deprived of monstrosity, she is a simulated other-than that marks the very indecisiveness of the norm. A fake Medea in the time of mimicry, displacing trauma and empowering a new woman, no longer monstrous, but certainly more scarred by the markings of an invisible and inbred pain.

Works Cited

Assmann, Jan. "Re-Membering Osiris: Vom Totenkult zur kulturellen Frinne rung." *ReMembering the Body*. Gabriele Brandstetter and Hortensia Völckers, eds. Ostfildem-Ruit: Hantje-Catz, 2000. 44–79.

Baudrillard, Jean. *L'Echange symbolique et la mort*. Paris: Seuil, 1976.

Baumann, Zygmunt. *Moderne undAmbivalenz*. Frankfurt am Main: Fischer, 1996.

Bell, Catherine. *Ritual Theory. Ritual Practice*. Oxford: OUP, 1992.

Bennet, Melba Berry. *The Stone Mason of Tor House: The Life and Work of Robinson Jeffers*. Los Angeles: The Ward Richie Press, 1966.

Blumenberg, Hans. *Arbeit am Mythos*. Frankfurt am Main: Suhrkamp, 1983.

Boswell, Jeanetta. *Robinson Jeffers and the Critics, 1912–1983: A Bibliography of Secondary Sources with Selective Annotations*. Metuchen, NJ and London: Scarecrow, 1986.

Braidotti, Rosi. *Nomadic Subjects*. New York: Columbia UP, 1994.

Bronfen, Elisabeth. *Over Her Dead Body. Death, Femininity and the Aesthetic*. Manchester: U of Manchester P, 1992.

Brophy, Robert J. "Jeffer's *Cawdor* and the Hippolytus Story." *Western American Literature* 7 (1973): 171–178.

Burkert, Walter. *Wilder Ursprung. Opferritual und Mythos bei den Griechen*. Berlin: Wagenbach, 1991.

Butler, Judith. *Gender Trouble*. London: Routledge, 1990.

Deleuze, Gilles. *Différence et repetition*. Paris: du Seuil, 1968.

Douglas, Mary. *Purity and Danger: An Analysis of the Concepts of Pollution and Taboo*. London: Routledge, 2001.

Euripides. Medea. Trans. Philip Vellacott. Harmondsworth: Penguin, 1983.

Fischbach, Ute. "Endlich Schluß mit der alten Lüge über Medea." *Münchner Merkur* Jan. 1 (1985): 22.

Fisher, Eva-Elisabeth. "Das Mitleid der Opfer." *Süddeutsche Zeitung*. Dec. 24 (1984): 125–6.

Foucault, Michel. *Omnis et singulatim: Towards a Critic of 'Political Reason'*. Salt Lake City: U of Utah P, 1988.

Frazer, James. *The Golden Bough*. 1922. Ware: Wordsworth, 1993.

Fritz, Kurt von. "Die Entwicklung der Iason-Medea Sage und die Medea des Euripides." *Antike und moderne Tragödie. Neun Abhandlungen*. Berlin: Walter de Gruyter & Co, 1962. 322–493.

Fühmann, Franz. "Das mythische Element in der Literatur." *Erfahrungen und Widersprüche. Versuche über Literatur*. Frankfurt am Main: Suhrkamp, 1976. 199–220.

Gascard, Johannes. *Medea-Morphosen. Eine mytho-psychohistorische Untersuchung zur Rolle des Mann-Weiblichen im Kulturprozess.* Berlin: Düncker und Humblot, 1993.

Girard, René. *Das Heilige und die Gewalt.* Frankfurt am Main: Fischer, 1984.

Grosz, Elizabeth. *Volatile Bodies. Toward a Corporeal Feminism.* Bloomington: Indiana UP, 1994.

Haraway, Donna. *Cyborgs and Women: The Reinvention of Nature.* London: Free Association Books, 1990

Hesse, Eva. "Die Exzesse von Robinson Jeffers." *Robinson Jeffers. Gedichte.* Passau: Andreas-Haller Verlag, 1984. 109–163.

Irigaray, Luce. *Ce sexe que n'est pas un.* Paris: du Seuil, 1977.

Jeffers, Robinson. *Cawdor and Medea.* New York: New Directions Books, 1977.

Johnston, Sarah Iles. "Corinthian Medea and the Cult of Hera Akraia." *Medea.* James J. Clauss and Sarah Iles Johnston, eds. Princeton: Princeton UP, 1997. 44–70.

Kamper, Dietmar. "Lektüre als Narbenschrift." *Transfigurationen des Körpers. Spuren der Gewalt in der Geschichte.* Berlin: de Gruyter, 1989. 1–7.

Kantorowicz, Emst. *Die zwei Körper des Königs. Eine Studie zur politischen Theologie des Mittelalters.* Munich: Beck, 1990.

Karman, James. *Robinson Jeffers. Poet of California.* Brownsville: Story Line Press, 1995.

Kerényi, Karl. "Medea." *Medea.* Joachim Schlöndorff, ed. Munich: Langen-Müller Verlag, 1963. 9–29.

Krevans, Nita. "Medea as Foundation-Heoine." *Medea.* James J. Clauss and Sarah Iles Johnston, eds. Princeton: Princeton UP, 1997. 71–82

Kristeva, Julia. *La révolution du language poétique.* Paris: du Seuil, 1974.

Lacan, Jacques. *Ecrits,* Paris: Seuil, 1966.

Laqueur, Thomas. *Making Sex. Body and Gender from the Greeks to Freud.* Cambridge, Mass: Harvard UP, 1990.

Lauretis, Teresa de. "Eccentric Subjects: Feminist Theory and Historical Consciousness." *Feminist Studies* 16: 1 (1990): 115–50.

Le Rider, Jacques. *Das Ende der Illusion. Zur Kritik der Moderne.* Vienna: ÖBV, 1990.

Lewis, Reina. *Gendering Orientalism. Race, Femininity and Representation.* London: Routledge, 1996.

Lowe, Lisa. "Nationalism and Exoticism: Nineteenth-Century Others in Flaubert's *Salammbô* and *L'Éducation sentimentale.*" *Macropolitics of Nineteenth-Century Literature: Nationalism, Exoticism, Imperialism.* Jonathan Arac and Harriet Ritvo, eds. Philadelphia: U of Pennsylvania P, 1991. 135–55.

Man, Paul de. *Allegories of Reading. Figural Language in Rousseau, Nietzsche, Rilke and Proust.* New Haven: Yale UP, 1979.

Nietzsche, Friedrich. *Genealogie der Moral.* Munich: dtv/de Gruyter, 1990.

Radtke, Peter. *M wie Tabori. Erfahrungen eines behinderten Schauspielers.* Zürich: Pendo, 1988.
Ranke Graves, Robert von. *Griechische Mythologie. Quellen und Deutung.* Reinbek bei Hamburg: Rowohlt, 1989.
Rich, Adrienne. *Blood, Bread and Poetry: Selected Prose 1979–1985.* London: Virago, 1987.
Rotschild, Thomas. "Die Wunde versteht das Messer. Juden auf Taboris Bühne." *Text + Kritik* 133 (1997): 4–9
Said, Edward. *Orientalism.* Harmondsworth: Penguin, 1978.
Tabori, George. *M*, (Unpublished manuscript) 1984.
Turner, Victor. *The Ritual Process: Structure and Anti-Structure.* Ithaca: Cornell UP, 1969.
Vardamis, Alex A. "Robinson Jeffers: Poet of Controversy." *Centennial Essays for Robinson Jeffers.* Robert Zaller, ed. Newark: U of Delaware P, 1991. 67–90.
Virilio, Paul. *L'art du moteur.* Paris: Galilée, 1993.

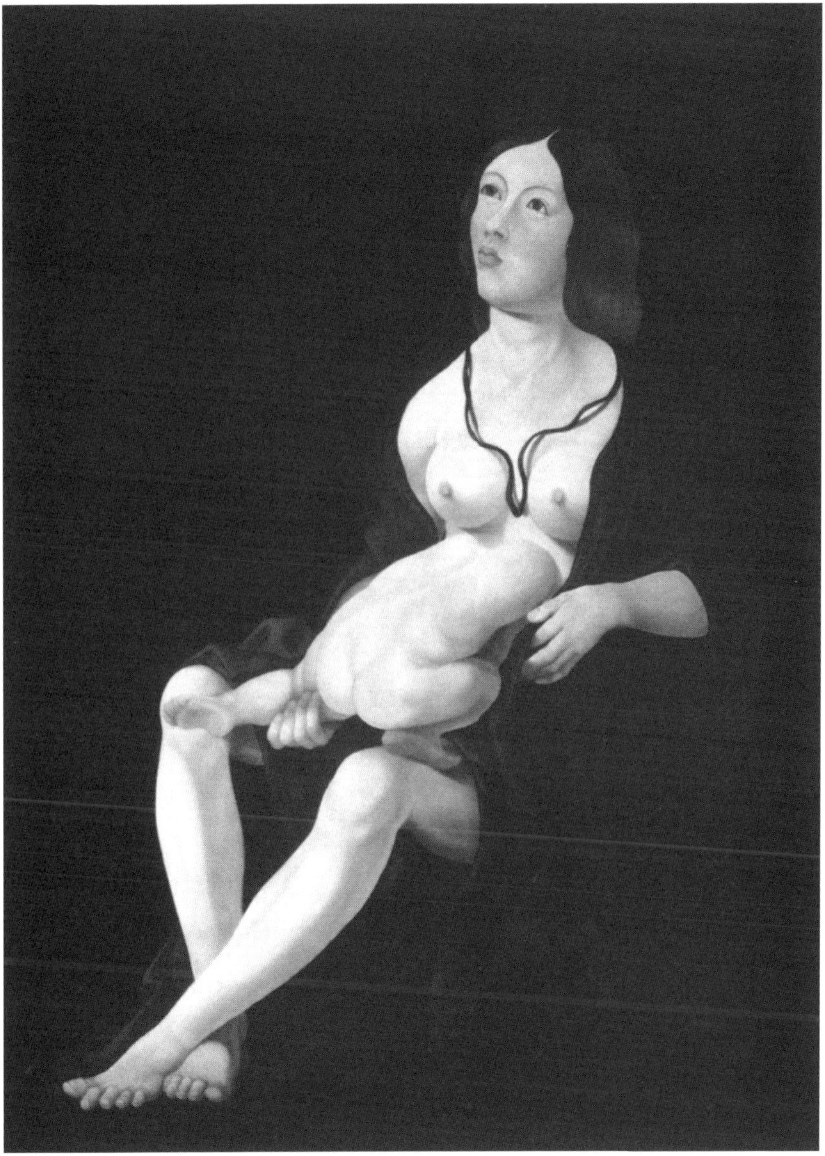

Marina Núñez. "Sin título (monstruas)" (Without title – monstresses)
Private Collection, Madrid, 1994.

Vitas

Kerstin Bergman has a Ph.D. in Comparative Literature from Lund University, Sweden. Currently she is studying the depiction of sense perceptions in contemporary literature and film, in a project financed by the Faculty of Humanities, Lund University. She is the author of *En möjlig värld: En tematisk studie av Lars Gustafssons 1990-talsromaner* ('A Concievable World: A Thematic Study of Lars Gustafsson's Novels from the 1990s,' Gidlunds 2002).

Ángel Cagigas. Graduate in Philosophy and Ph.D. in Psychology from the University of Salamanca. He is currently teaching History of Psychology as Associate Profesor at the University of Jaén. He is the Director of Ediciones Lunar and has written a great variety of articles and books, among which *Genio y figura*, *Georg Groddeck: el soñador de mundos*, *Guía de viaje por una historia de la psicología*, and *La histeria de Charcot* should be mentioned.

Isabel Capeloa Gil, born in 1965, is Professor of German Studies at the Catholic University of Portugal. Ph.D. thesis: *Mythographies. Figurations of Antigone, Cassandra and Medea in German 20th Century Drama*. Her publications include work on intermedia studies, particularly dance and literature, women's studies and 20th century drama. Her forthcoming book is *What is Postfeminism?* (2004)

Valérie de Courville Nicol is Assistant Professor of Sociology at the University of Concordia in Montreal. Her research interests include fear and risk, popular literature, and studies in governmentality. She has published articles on gothic literature and on fear and modern subjectivity, and has a book forthcoming, *Le soupçon gothique*. She is currently conducting research on self-help books with a focus on disorders of fear.

Dana Milstein teaches World Literature of Ancient and Modern Civilization for the English Department at Baruch College, City University of New York. She has published and presented articles devoted primarily to fin-de-siècle Europe, and on theoretical topics including space and time in Oriental and Western culture, and the effect of venereal disease upon creativity. She is currently writing a book-length work devoted to Debussy and the transposition of the Arts in Modern Europe. Dana is also a singer and songwriter. Her music can be accessed at www.daynblakeley.com.

Mark Mossman is Assistant Professor of English at Western Illinois University. His teaching interests include poetry, 19th century British Literature and Culture. He has recently published on Mary Lamb, Elizabeth Gaskell, Mary Shelley, and visible disability in the college classroom. He is currently working on an essay concerning Rousseau, Samuel Johnson, the Shelleys, and the origin of disability.

Marina Núñez is an internationally known Spanish painter. So far her work has centred on the representation of the female body as victim and marked subject. Recently her interest is geared towards cyborgs as metaphors of abjection and hybridity.

Nieves Pascual is Associate Professor of North American Literature at the University of Jaén in Spain. She has published *El otro oficio de los profesores: la novela universitaria anglo-americana*, and has co-authored: *Otras literaturas en lengua inglesa: una alternativa crítica*. Currently she is working on a manuscript on hunger and women's writing.

Markus Rheindorf is Junior Fellow at the International Research Centre for Cultural Studies in Vienna and is currently working on his Ph.D. thesis: 'A Cultural History of Early Film Theory', at the University of Vienna and the Amsterdam School of Cultural Analysis. He also teaches media and discourse analysis at the

University of Vienna. His research interests are largely transdisciplinary and include discourse analysis, semiotics, film theory and cultural studies. He has published a number of articles on popular culture and post-modern theory on such diverse topics as the literary fantastic in comics, the film adaptations of video games and the holistic poetics of Paul Auster.

Eluned Summers-Bremmer is Lecturer in Women's Studies at the University of Auckland, New Zealand, where she teaches gender and sexuality in the history of sciences and the arts and media. She has published in such journals as *New Formations, Hypatia* and *Feminist Studies*, and in numerous edited collections, and she is currently at work on two book-length projects, one on the function of memory in the imagination and the other on the contemporary function of the fantasy of childhood.

Rossana Zaera graduated in Applied Arts in Castellón. In 1988 she opened a successful workshop to teach design. Her work has been exhibited in different parts of the country. Zaera has been the recipient of numerous prestigious awards.